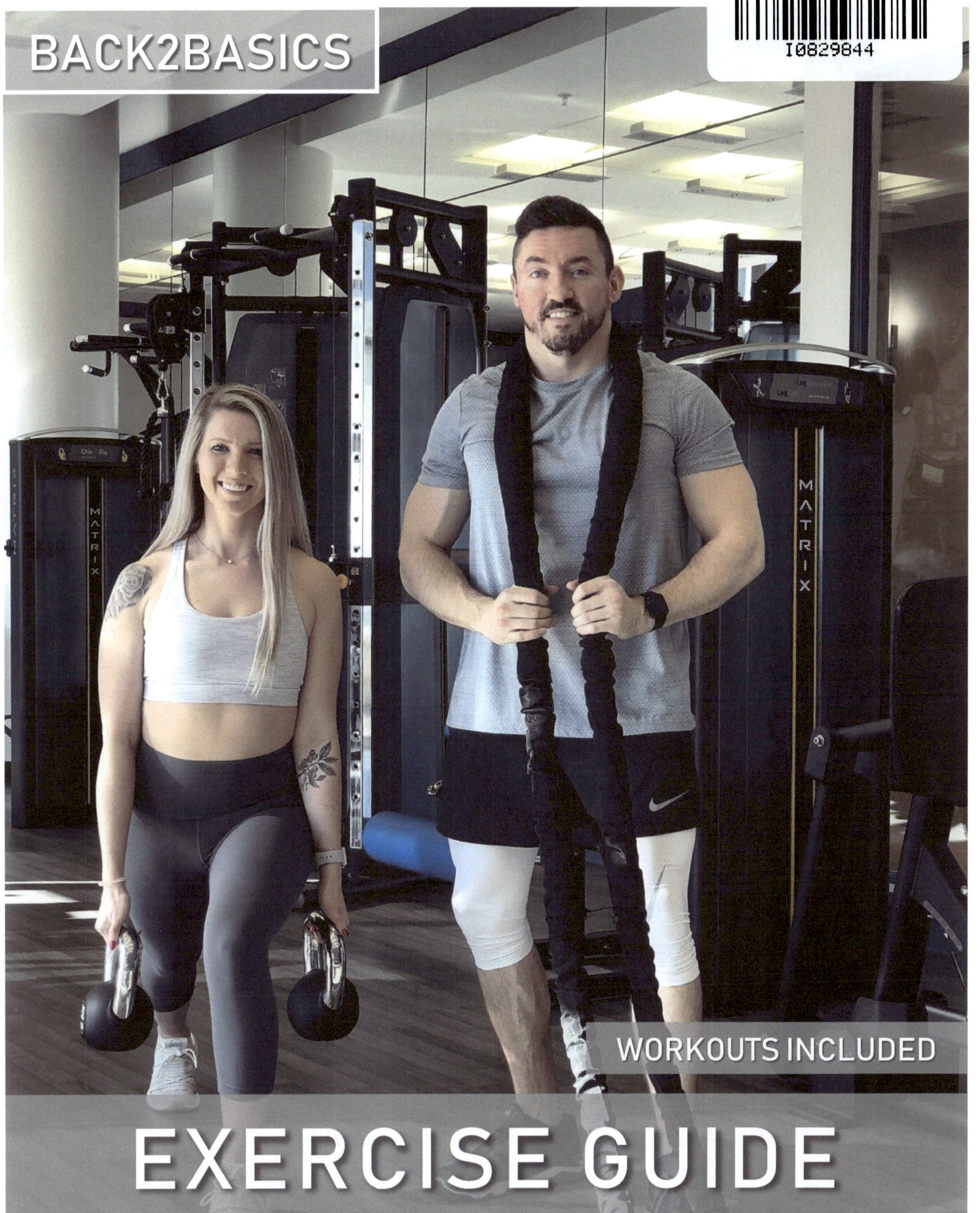
BACK2BASICS
I0829844
WORKOUTS INCLUDED
EXERCISE GUIDE
The Basics of Exercise For Improving Your Health

TABLE OF CONTENTS

Here's what you can find within this guide:

INTRODUCTION

Fitness is the condition of being healthy, being physically fit, being able to function properly as the human body was intended. Exercise is intended to improve our fitness.

EVERY HUMAN BODY NEEDS EXERCISE

Hi, I'm Doug. This is me

I'm a lifelong fitness enthusiast, personal trainer, group fitness instructor, gym owner, nutrition expert, and former athlete. I live and breath fitness, and I want to help others enhance their lives by adopting a healthier lifestyle.

I've worked with hundreds of individuals on their fitness, each with unique goals and challenges. There isn't a "one size fits all" plan when it comes to your health. With so much misinformation being marketed for fitness fads and quick-fix workouts, it's difficult to tell what really works and what you should be doing.

I developed this guide to explain how exercise fundamentally works, how it impacts your body, and how you can take the best approach for meeting your individual health and fitness goals.

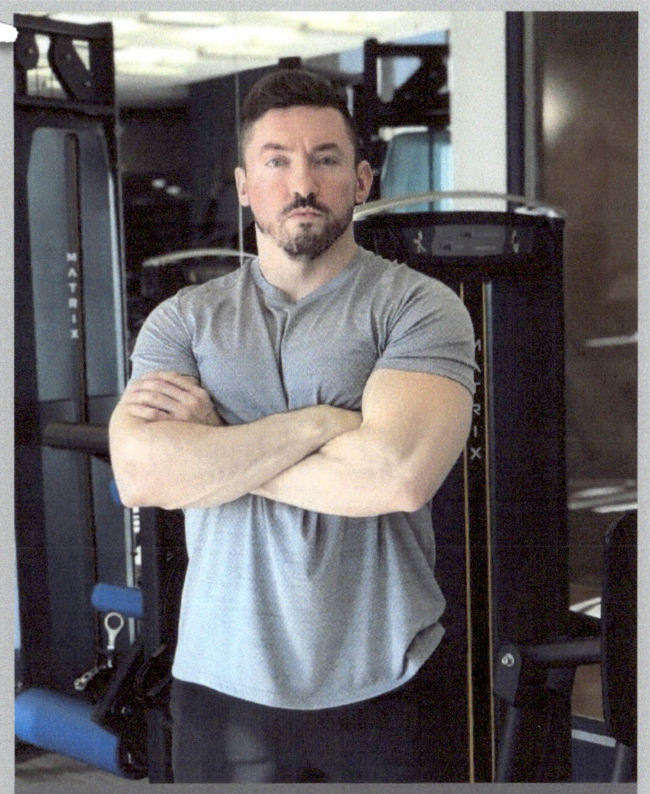

Doug's Exercise Principles:

1. Every body needs exercise
2. Not all exercise is created equally
3. Short-term approaches will give you short-term benefits
4. The impacts of exercise are equivalent to the effort you put in

QUICK REFERENCES

First things first, let's get an understanding of the body and some key terms used in fitness. It may not make sense initially, but it'll all come together, I promise!

BODY COMPOSITION

Your body composition is more than your appearance, it is the makeup of fat vs fat-free mass (muscle, bone, water, organs, etc.) on your body. A healthy body composition is one that has a lower percentage of body fat (not to be confused with weight). Your body needs some fat to protect internal organs, store fuel for energy, regulate body hormones, but high percentages of body fat can lead to serious health disorders. Different forms of exercise can impact your body composition in different ways (e.g. burning fat, building muscle).

HEALTHY MALE
BODY COMPOSITION

Description	Bodyfat %
Essential	2 – 5 %
Athlete	6 – 13 %
Fit	14 – 17 %
Average	18 – 24 %
Obese	25 % +

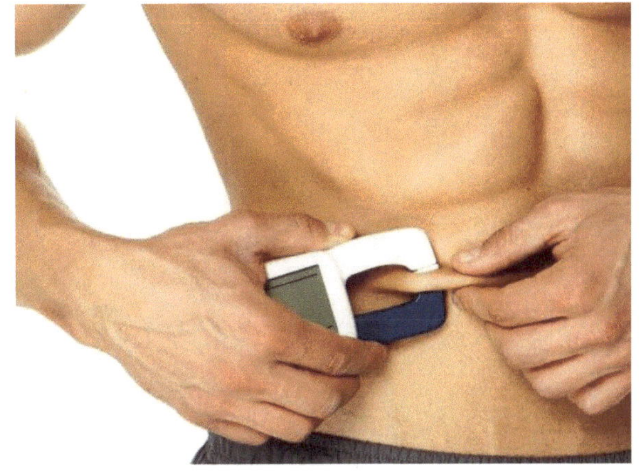

HEALTHY FEMALE
BODY COMPOSITION

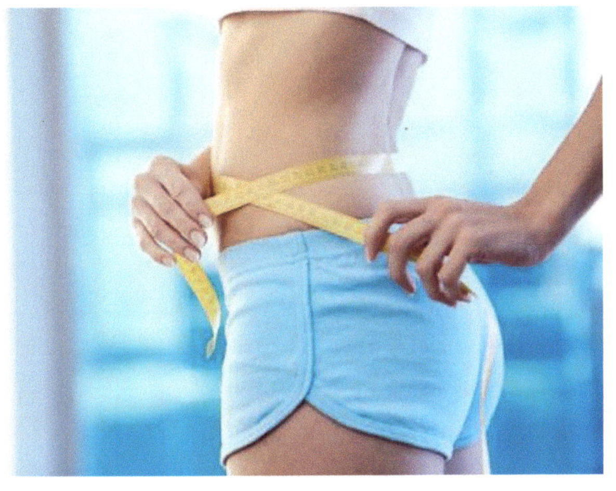

Description	Bodyfat %
Essential	10 – 13 %
Athlete	14 – 20 %
Fit	21 – 24 %
Average	25 – 31 %
Obese	32 % +

Your individual body type can also impact your body composition (see next page).

BODY TYPES

Your genetics primarily dictate your general body shape and body type. Your body type can influence what type of exercise your body needs and responds to. Below are the 3 high-level body types:

1. **Ectomorph:** Generally lean and elongated bodies which may have difficulty building muscle mass.
2. **Mesomorph:** Muscular / athletic physique with low bodyfat, high metabolism and responsive muscles.
3. **Endomorph:** Generally bigger and rounder ("curvy") with a higher tendency to store bodyfat.

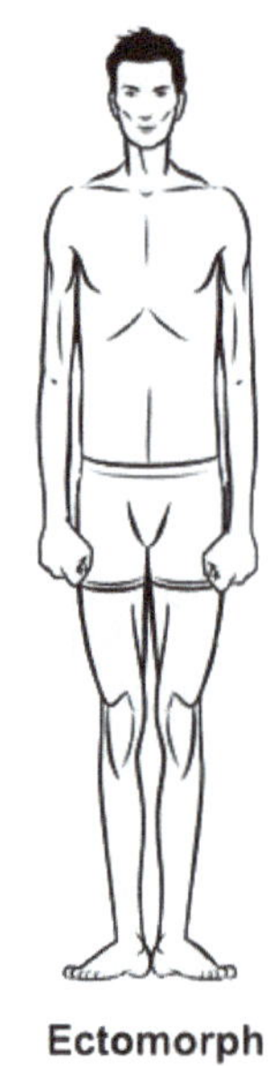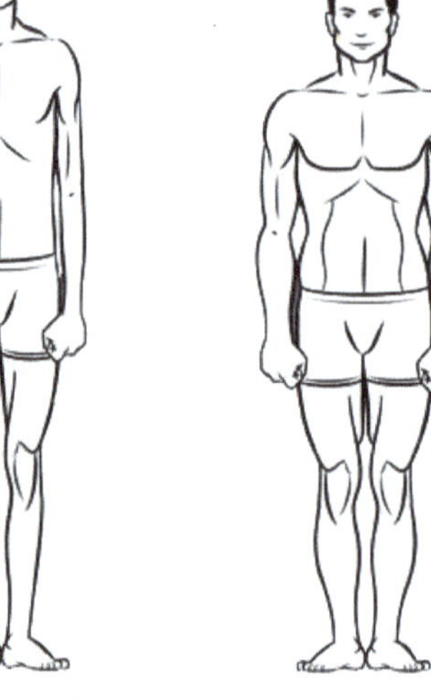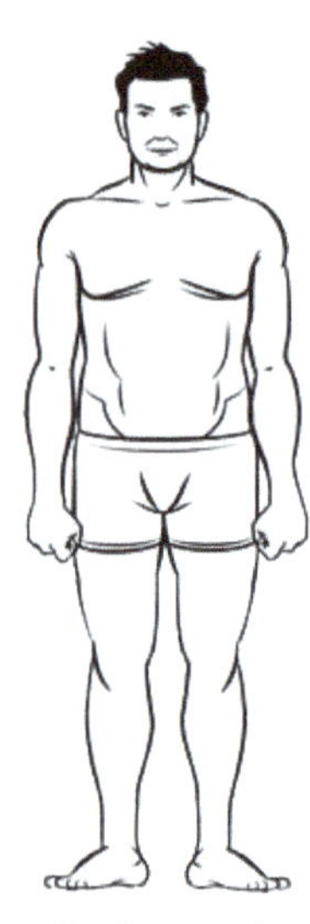

Ectomorph   Mesomorph   Endomorph

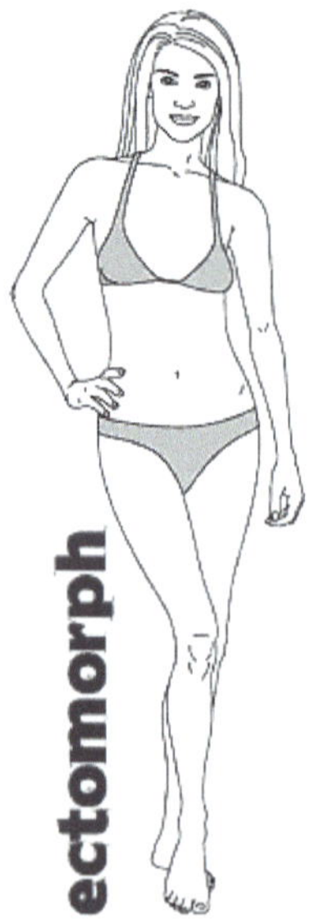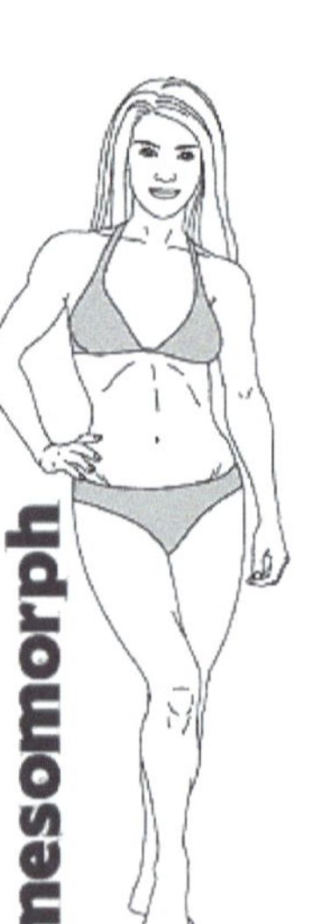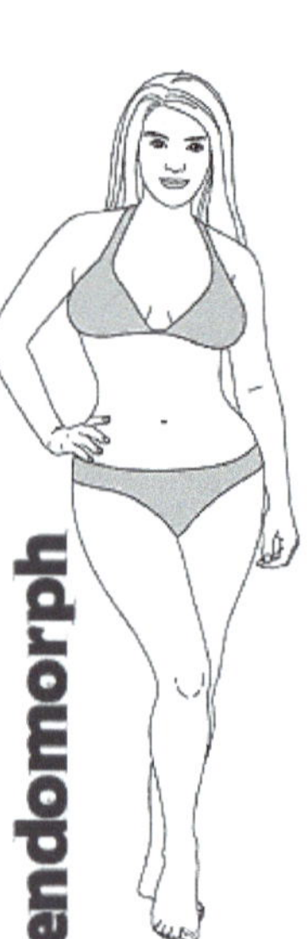

MUSCLE DIAGRAM

Regardless of body type, every body has muscle. There are 650+ muscles in the human body. Below are the major muscle groups used in exercise:

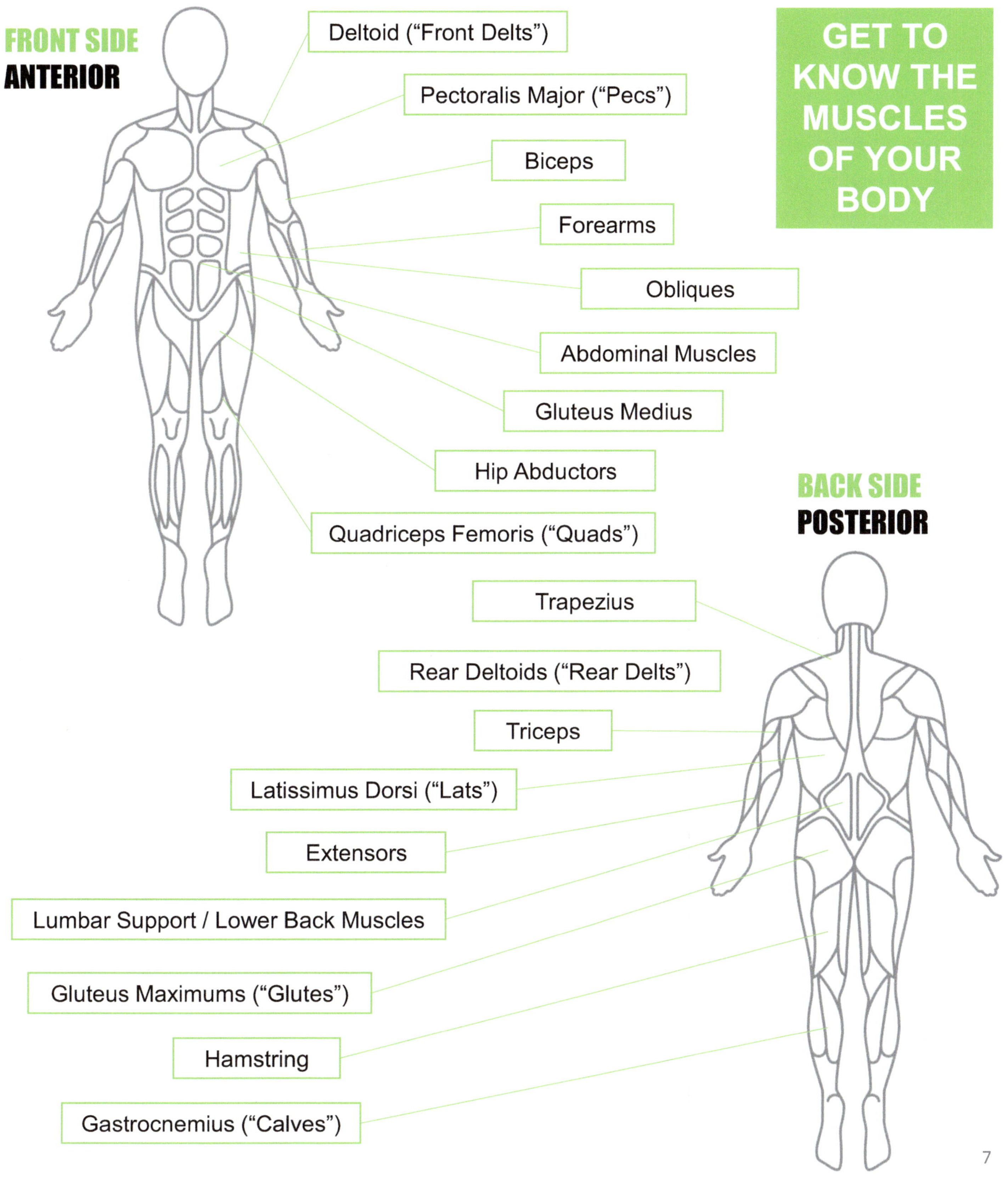

Below are some of the terms we'll be discussing throughout this guide.

Don't worry, you don't need to memorize them. We'll discuss many of them in context later on.

KEY WORD DEFINITIONS

Aerobic Exercise – Activity intended to improve the body's cardiovascular system (endurance). This is all about breathing, blood flow and elevating the heart rate.

Anaerobic Exercise – Activity that requires intense exertion in a short period of time. This is used to promote strength, speed, power and muscle mass.

Body Composition - The makeup of the body in terms of lean mass (muscle, bone, vital tissue and organs) and fat mass. An optimal ratio of fat to lean mass is an indication of physical fitness.

Fat – A type of nutrient used for fuel (energy) and to help your body absorb vitamins. The body can store excess/unwanted fat depending upon food consumption and activity levels.

Muscle – Soft tissue on the body that performs to produce force and motion (and can burn fat).

Muscular Strength - Ability of a muscle to exert force for a brief period of time. This can be measured by the level of resistance or weight used in an exercise.

Muscular Endurance - The ability of a muscle, or a group of muscles, to sustain repeated contractions or to continue applying force. This is how long your muscles can last.

Flexibility/Mobility - The ability to move joints freely and use muscles through their full intended range of motion.

Repetitions (Reps) – A repetition is one complete motion of an exercise. We generally perform exercises in several repetitions. If you perform 10 squats in a row, it would be considered 10 reps.

Sets – A set is a group of consecutive repetitions. If you performed 10 reps of a squat, then took a breather and performed 10 more reps, then you will have completed 2 sets. A workout plan will indicate how many sets and reps you'll perform of each exercise.

Circuit – A series of exercises performed back to back. In a circuit, you'll perform an exercise for a number of repetitions immediately followed by the next exercise in the circuit for a number of repetitions (ex: 1 set of 10 pushups, 10 situps, then 10 squats).

Resistance Training – Use of resistance to workout the body (primary form of anaerobic training).

High Intensity Interval Training (HIIT) – Executing short bursts of highly intense exercise (to increase capacity), followed by short periods of rest/recovery.

Metabolism – The range of chemical processes that occur that keep you alive, by burning Calories for fuel.

(Basel) Metabolic Rate – The amount of Calories required to keep your body functioning at rest / the amount of Calories your body will burn at rest.

THE BASICS OF EXERCISE

Let's talk about why exercise is important, the different forms of exercise, and what might work best for your body.

Your Body Needs Exercise

The two things that (literally) keep your body alive are physical activity and consumption of nutrients. Without those two things your body cannot function.

Physical activity is any movement carried out by the muscles that requires energy. Our bodies can get physical activity from things like walking through the grocery store, throwing a ball with our kids, or walking up a flight of stairs.

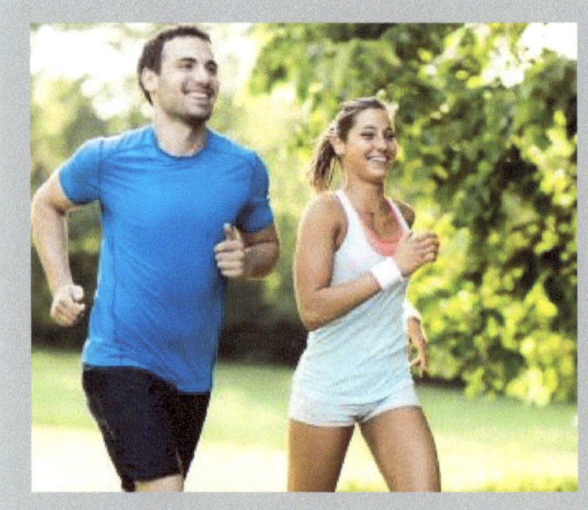

Exercise, is planned, structured and intentional movement (activity) intended to improve or maintain your health and fitness.

General activity keeps our body alive (status quo), exercise makes our body more efficient, more resilient, and more "fit" for life (more healthy).

Here are just a few of the benefits of dedicated exercise:

- maintaining a healthy body composition
- reducing risk of disease, illness and injury
- enhancing memory and cognitive function
- improving mental health and mood
- strengthening muscles and bones
- increasing your energy levels and focus
- relieving stress
- promoting better sleep

FUNDAMENTALS OF EXERCISE

How does Exercise work?

Exercise is performed through dedicated movement that increases blood flow and oxygen to your tissue, elevates your heart rate, engages muscles and activates motor function. Exercise requires your body to put in extra work. That extra work is what brings on the health benefits. Here's how some of it works:

Burning Calories - When your body puts in work, it requires energy, which comes from Calories. Those Calories come from our consumption of foods. Burning more Calories then we consume is how we lose weight.

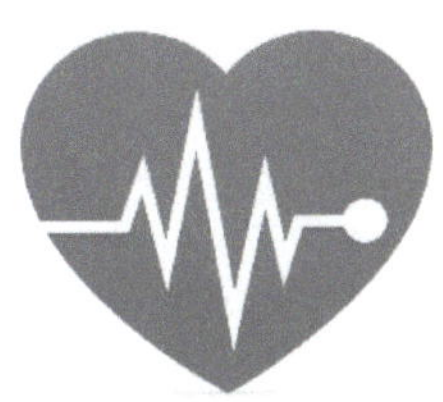

Improving Body Functions – The extra workload put on our body from exercise overtime teaches our body how to perform its functions better and more efficiently (from walking to breathing to metabolizing). The more your exercise, the better your body gets at its functions.

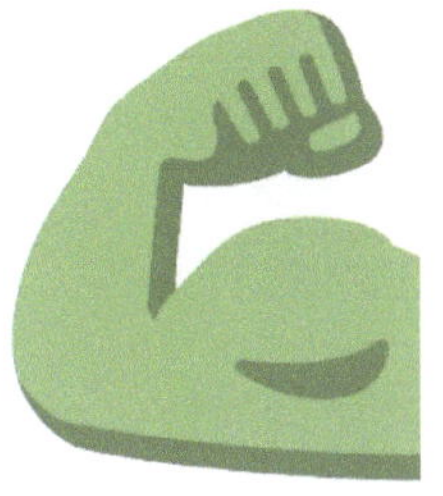

Muscle Growth – During exercise while muscles are challenged, the muscle fibers break down. Your body responds by repairing these fibers to make them stronger by increasing size or amount of fibers (thus enhancing your body composition). The more muscle you have, the higher your metabolism (ability to burn Calories) will be.

There are many ways to exercise

There are several different forms of exercise, and several different ways to execute the same forms of exercise. Depending upon what components of your body the exercise works, the benefits to your body will vary. Not all exercise is created equally and different approaches to exercise may yield better results for each individual.

Exercise can be segmented into two major categories:

Aerobic Exercise (Cardio) and **Anaerobic Exercise**

AEROBIC EXERCISE

Aerobic Exercise (Cardio)

Aerobic training methods are general movements at a low to moderate intensity for extended periods of time. They primarily work your cardiovascular system (your heart), by requiring increased oxygen and blood. Cardio exercise will elevate your heart rate while increasing blood flow and oxygen to the muscles, enabling your body to sweat and burn Calories. This process helps your body utilize oxygen more efficiently, increasing your endurance / conditioning. The Calorie burn throughout cardio exercise can be beneficial when your goal is to lose weight.

Popular Forms of Cardio Training

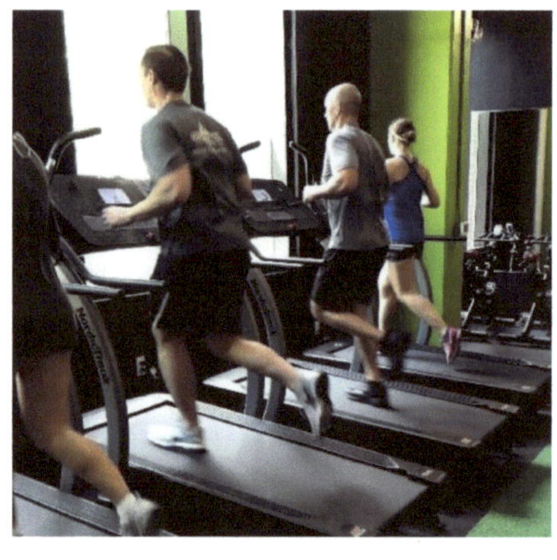

- Running / Jogging
- Biking / Spinning
- Rowing
- Aerobics Classes
- Elliptical Training

Cardio can be done almost anywhere, and doesn't require much skill, so it's an easy go-to for most individuals. Though cardio can be great for shedding weight, it has minimal impact on re-shaping your body or building muscle mass (body composition).

Cardio Recommendation 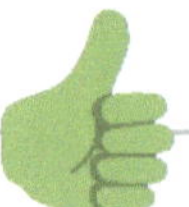

Cardiovascular exercise should be a part of every fitness plan, but it should not be the only type of activity performed. The frequency and duration of cardio should depend on several factors, but a general recommendation for adults would be to perform moderate intensity cardio 2-3x per week for 30 minutes.

ANAEROBIC EXERCISE

Anaerobic Exercise

Anaerobic training methods involve short intense bursts of physical activity where the body uses energy stored in your muscles, as opposed to relying on oxygen. These exercises work your muscles to strengthen and tone your body, enhance performance, and burn fat. Anaerobic exercise can also help shed pounds when done with high intensity.

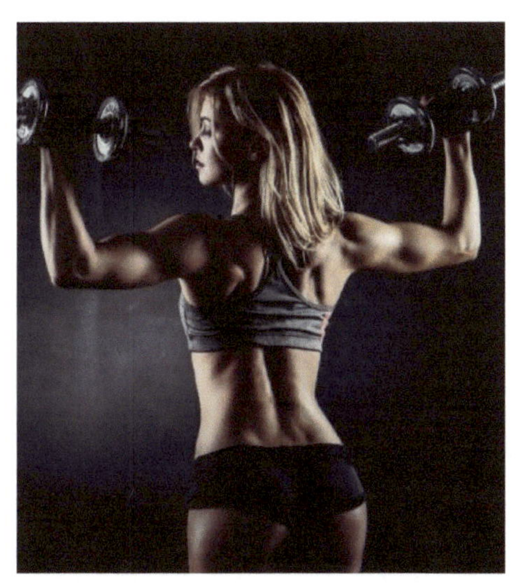

Popular Forms of Anaerobic Training

- **Resistance Training** – Use of resistance to work your muscles, generally via the use of weights, but can also be done with bodyweight (calisthenics) and other tools.

- **High Intensity Interval Training** – Using short periods to push yourself to capacity at high intensity, followed by rest periods.

- **Plyometrics** – Dynamic exercises in which muscles exert maximum force (e.g., jumping).

Developing muscle does NOT necessarily mean becoming big and bulky. Every body has and needs muscle. Resistance training helps develop **lean muscle** which has a TON of benefits for your body, including actively burning fat (body composition).

Anaerobic Recommendation

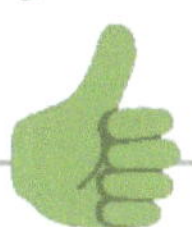

Resistance training should be a part of every fitness routine. Incorporating other methods of anaerobic exercise depends upon your skill level and goals. For adults, a general recommendation is to perform moderate to high-intensity resistance training 2-4x per week for 45 minutes or more.

IMPACT TO YOUR BODY

Since the two methods use your body in different ways, they have a different impact on your body composition.

Aerobic Body Composition Impact

During cardio, while energy is expended (Calories) it can lead to weight loss. That weight loss could come from fat or muscle depending upon the duration and frequency of cardio, your consumption of foods (like proteins), and more. Muscles are active during cardio so depending upon the factors on the previous page, cardio exercise could lead to some muscle development, but generally is not effective for re-shaping the body or building muscle mass. It may reduce your size but not change your overall shape or composition.

Anaerobic Body Composition Impact

Anaerobic exercises break down the muscles to rebuild them stronger, smarter, faster, and higher performing. During anaerobic exercise you're also expending energy (Calories) which can lead to weight loss. The development of muscle however can keep your bodyweight consistent, but will provide a healthier body composition (fat to muscle ratio). The more lean muscle you have on your body, the more fat your body will actively burn.

Don't Forget: Your body type and your genetics play a big role in how your body composition is impacted by different forms of exercise.

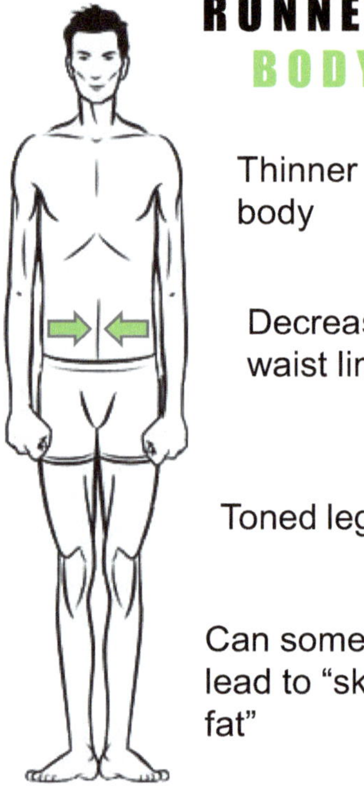

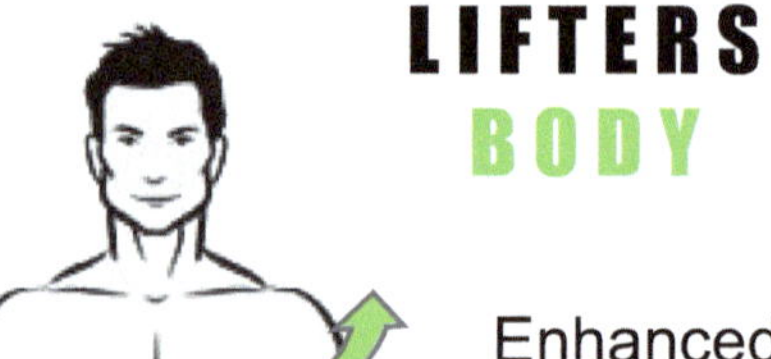

CHANGING THE OUTCOME

The way you perform exercises can change it's outcome.

Aerobic and anaerobic exercise do not have to be mutually exclusive, and every exercise doesn't have to fit into a category, but it's important to know what the exercise is intended to work on your body, and how to perform the exercise for the best outcome. You could add high-intensity to a cardio based exercise, such as turning jogging into sprints for anaerobic effects, and you could perform resistance exercises at a fast pace with minimal breaks to gain cardio benefits.

Below are some of the factors that influence the outcome and effectiveness of exercise:

- **Type of exercise** – which bodily component(s) the exercise works and how (the intention of the exercise)

- **Frequency of exercise** – how often you exercise (within a given week)

- **Duration of exercise** – time period you will perform the exercise for

- **Duration of rest periods** – time period you will rest for (within an individual workout as well as between workouts)

- **Set and rep schemes** – number of repetitions (reps) of each exercise and how many sets of reps you'll perform within a workout

- **Level of resistance** – how much weight, resistance, tension is applied

- **Level of intensity** – amount of effort / intensity applied to the exercise

Outside of exercise, there are external factors that can influence how your body individually responds to exercise, including:

- Your body type (see quick reference)
- Your genetics
- Your exercise history
- Your sleep, rest, and stress levels
- Your eating habits

Not All Exercise Is Created Equally

CHALLENGE & VARIETY

Step Out of Your Comfort Zone

The whole premise of exercise is based around making your body put in extra work. The challenge of that extra work is what makes it expend more energy and learn to perform better. If an exercise is easy, it's likely not requiring much work from your body, and therefore is not going to change you or improve your health. Exercise needs to be challenging in order to make an impact. The soreness you feel after a workout, is your body putting in the work to recover stronger (it's a good thing).

> *"If it doesn't challenge you, it doesn't change you"*

Your Body Needs Variety

The more you do something, the better your body gets at it. Our bodies are smart, they learn and adapt. However, if you do the same thing frequently and consistently enough, your body gets used to it, and it requires less from your body. At that point the impact and benefits of that exercise to your body decrease. When we stop seeing benefits of our work, this is what we call a "plateau". Your body needs change, something that makes it put in extra work; something to challenge it again.

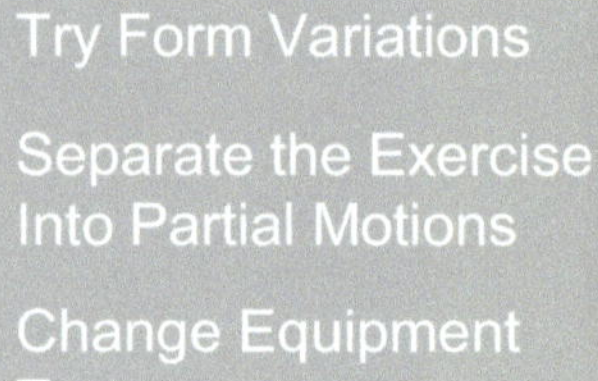
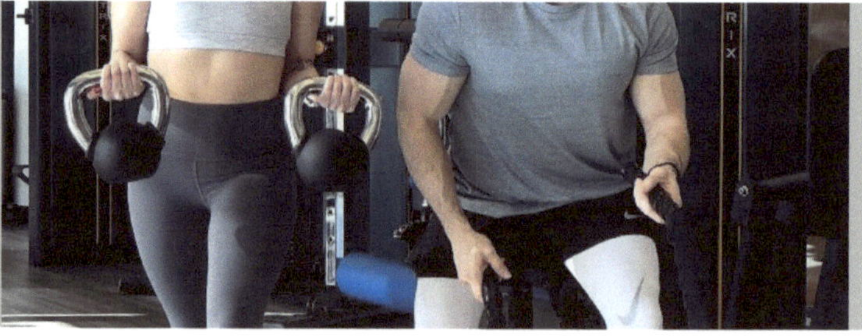

Variety can come in many forms. It can be as simple as adjusting the specific form of a motion, adjusting the rep scheme, or adjusting the resistance / intensity level. It can be as complicated as changing up your entire routine, daily, weekly, or monthly. The variety has to be enough to challenge your body (see above) to put in that extra work.

A COMPREHENSIVE APPROACH

Your body needs Aerobic and Anaerobic Exercise

Both methods have their pros and cons, but a combination of both cardiovascular exercise and anaerobic training will provide the most comprehensive approach to your health and produce the best results. There is no single exercise method that will provide everything your body needs. Your body needs variety and challenge in order to perform at its best.

CARDIO
Aerobic Exercise

Strengthens the heart and lungs:

- A strong cardiovascular system can lead to an extended life
- Higher endurance means breathing comes easier.

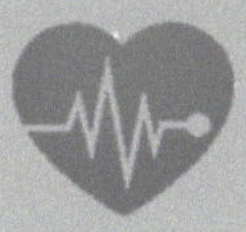

RESISTANCE
Anaerobic Exercise

Helps build lean muscle mass:

- Calories are burned more efficiently in bodies that have more muscle.
- Performing general physical activities becomes easier.

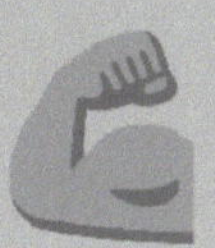

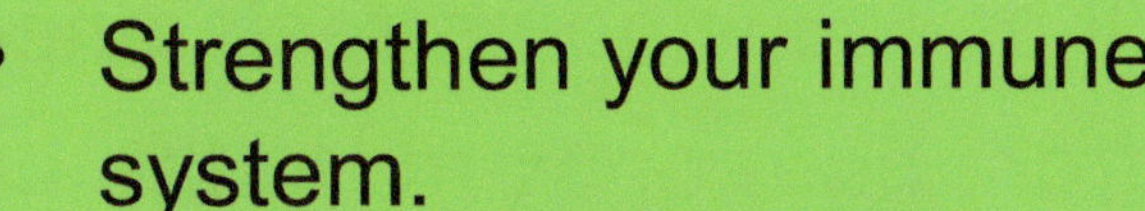

BOTH

- Strengthen your immune system.
- Improve your mood
- Enhance your focus and memory
- Improve your quality of life
- Maintain/control bodyweight

Key takeaways from this section:

- Exercise is about keeping our body active, moving, and functioning properly.

- Exercise has significant benefits to your health, outside of physical appearance.

- There are two major forms of exercise:
    - Aerobic - cardio based exercise (heart and breathing); best for building endurance and losing general weight.
    - Anaerobic - strength / functional based exercise (muscle); best for enhancing performance and body composition.

- There are several factors that influence the impact of exercise to your individual body.

- Some forms of exercise may yield different results for different people (based on genetics, body type, and outside factors).

- A comprehensive and challenging approach to fitness will produce the best results.

What's Next:

Since aerobic (or cardiovascular training) methods are fairly simple to execute, we'll be focusing on resistance training and anaerobic movement from here onward. In the next section, we're going to take a look at some basic functional movements that any body should be able to perform.

BASIC FUNCTIONAL MOVEMENTS

These are basic movements used in exercise (and in everyday life) that your body should be able to perform properly. These are the pushes, pulls, hinges, and rotations that are imperative to proper movement. These should be staples of an exercise routine.

Lower Body
Functional Motions

1 SQUAT

A pressing motion with the legs that requires just about every muscle group in the lower body, as well as some above (e.g. core). Think about these as taking a seat, without the chair.

- Stand with your feet hip width apart, guide your hips back then let your butt sit downward towards your heels.
- Your knees will bend and you'll want to make sure that they do not extend beyond the toes.
- You'll also want your upper body to remain upright as much as possible, don't let the shoulders extend past the knees (keep shoulders back and chest high).
- Drive upward through your heels to end back upright in the standing position.

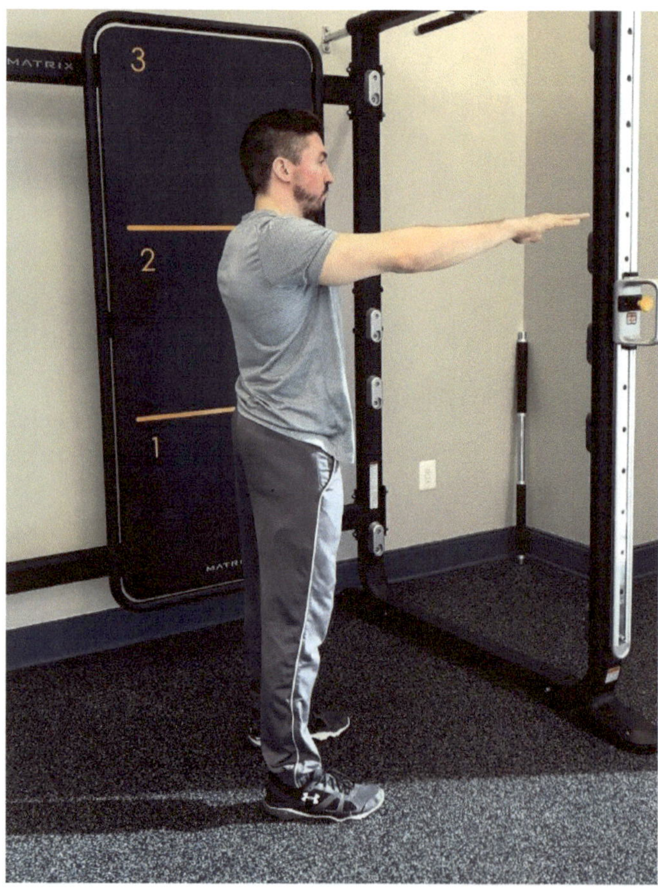
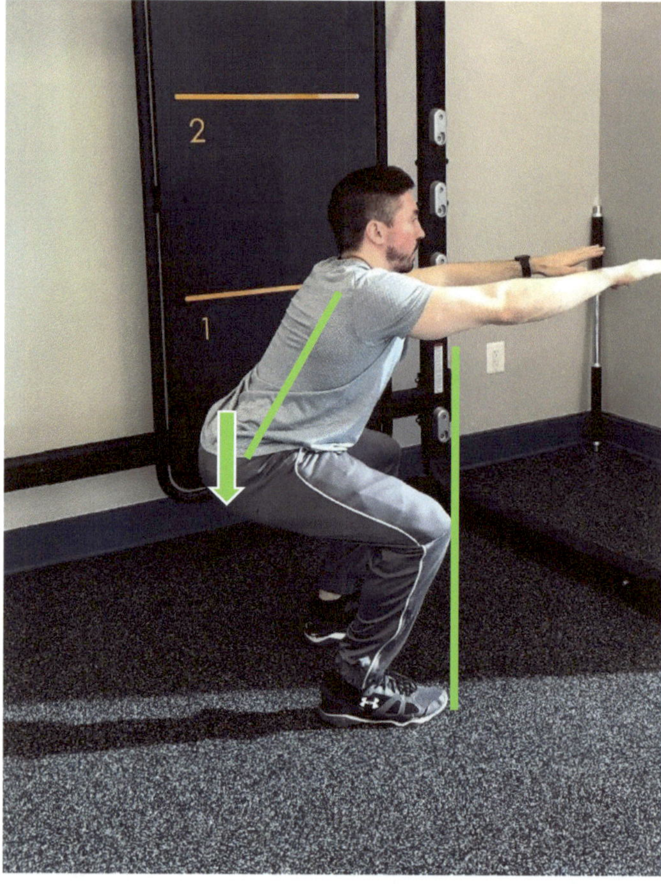

A squat is the motion that should generally be used when picking up objects from the ground, so you use your legs for strength not your back.

Lower Body
Functional Motions Cont'd

2 LUNGE

A bending motion with the legs that requires balance and coordination in addition to strength.

- Start out standing with your feet together, then pickup one foot and drive it forward while the other stays in place.
- Both knees should bend through the motion. The back knee should bend down towards the ground with the leg at a 90 degree angle, and the front knee should extend forward with the leg at a 90 degree angle.
- Don't let the front knee extend over the toes.
- Bring the front leg back to the starting position (keeping your back leg planted) to end the motion.

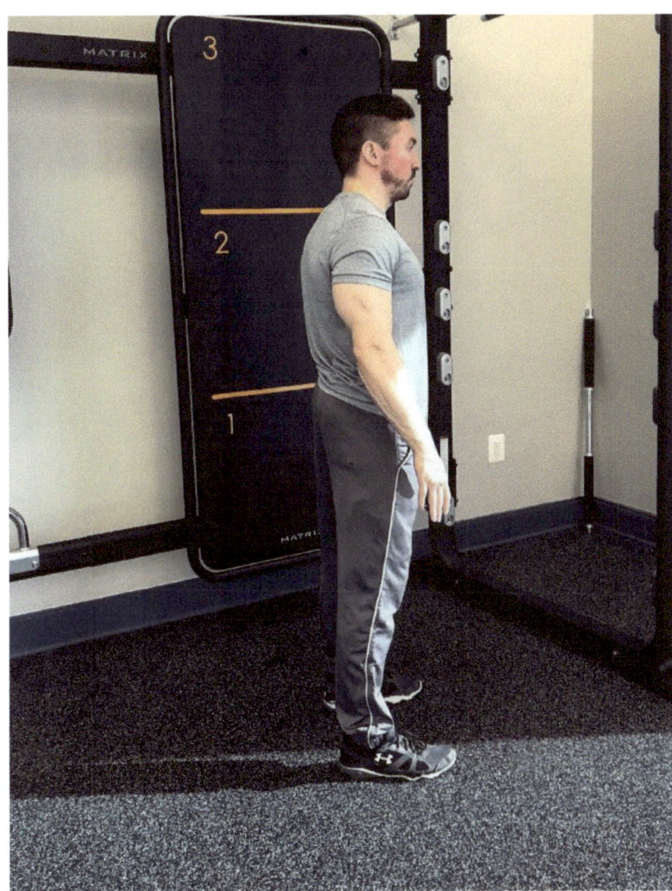
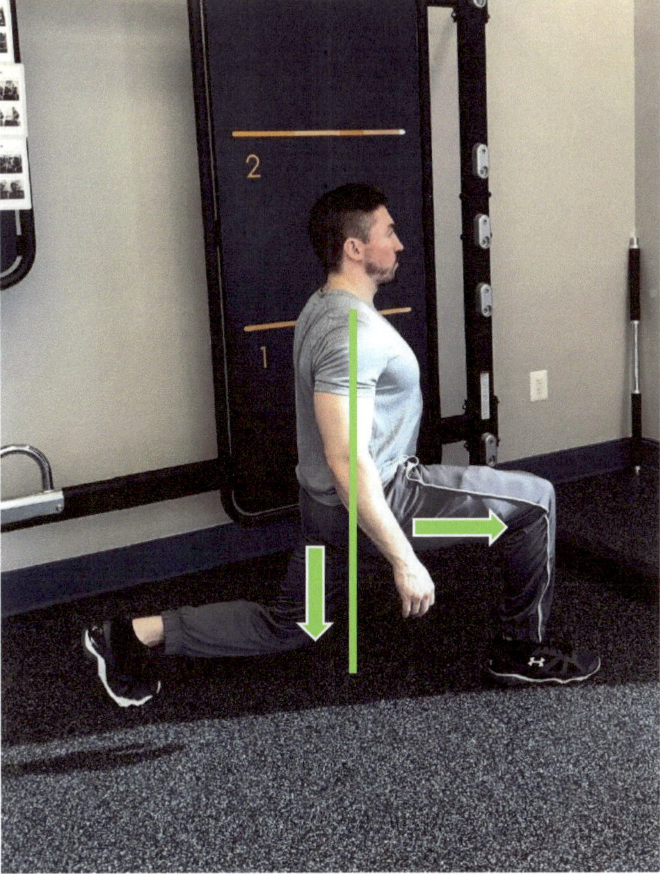

You should also be able to perform a reverse lunge (taking a leg backward) as well as a side lunge (taking a leg out to the side), but we'll stick to the basics for now.

Lower Body
Functional Motions Cont'd

3 DEADLIFT

A pulling motion with the legs (glutes and hamstrings) and hinging motion with the hips that engages several muscles groups in the lower body and the core at once.
- Stand with your feet hip width apart.
- Shoot your hips backward and let your chest come down forward at the same time.
- Allow your knees to slightly bend as your hips go backward and you slide your hands down the front side of your legs.
- On the way back up, drive upward through your heels, then thrust your hips forward.

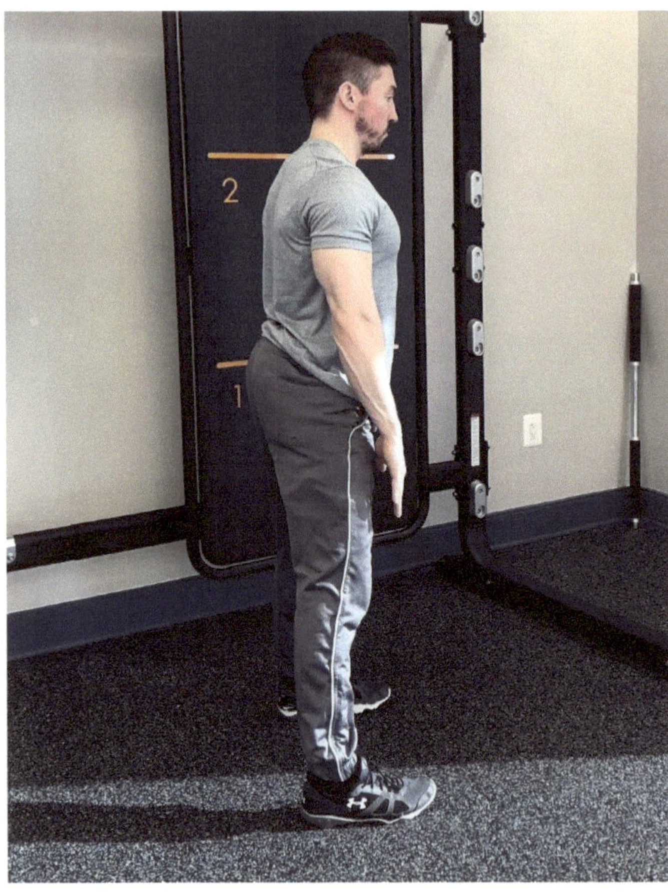
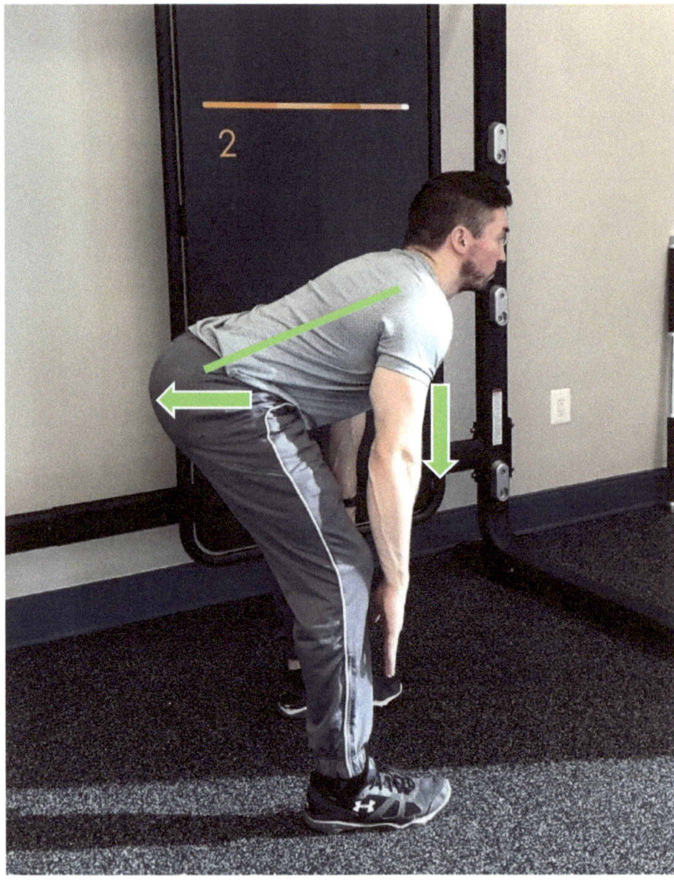

Focus on ensuring the hips go backward and your back remains in a straight line (not arched downwards) through the motion before adding weights. When using weights, keep them as close to your legs as possible.

Upper Body
Functional Motions

1 CHEST PRESS (PUSH-UP)

A forward pushing motion from the upper body primarily using the chest, shoulders, and arms. In this example, we'll be performing a bodyweight push-up.

- Start with your feet and hands on the ground with your body in a straight line (also known as the "high plank" position).
- Place your hands shoulder width apart, and place your feet together.
- Bend at your elbows and allow your whole body to descend downward.
- Ensure your body stays in a straight line by keeping your hips in line with your back throughout the full movement.
- Once you've bent your elbows to a 90 degree angle, propel your body upward by driving through your hands.

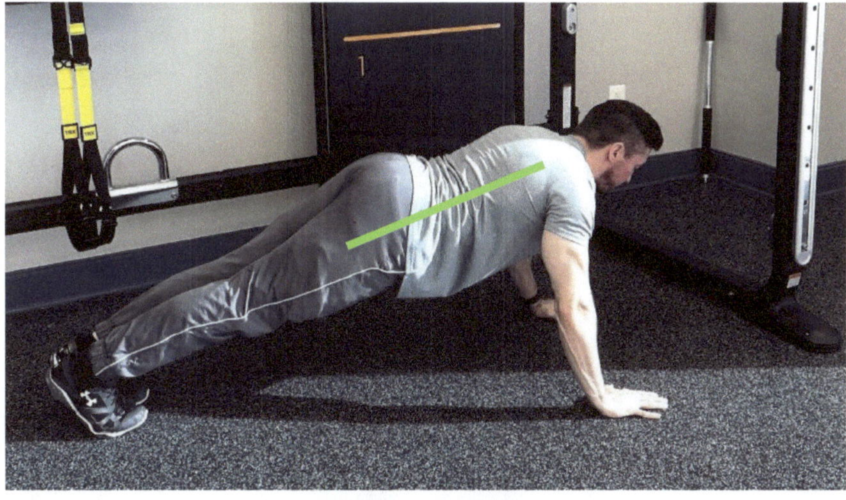

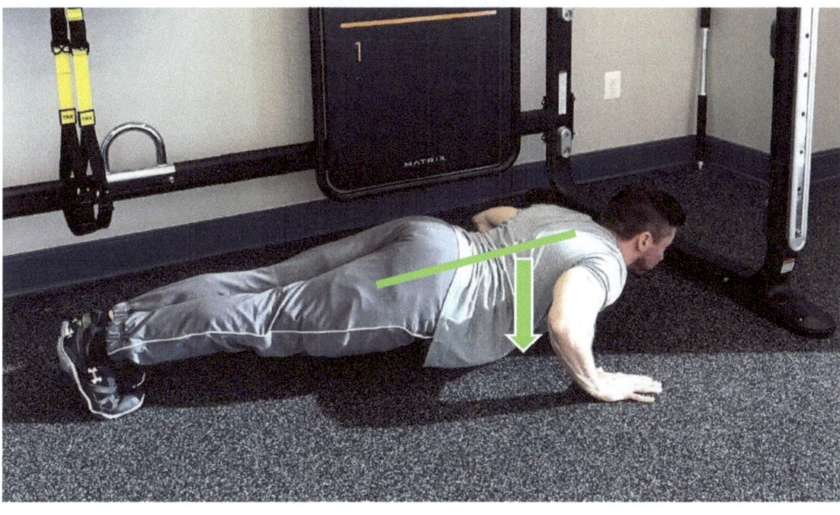

If a push-up is to difficult from this position, you can drop to your knees (both feet and knees remain on the ground) and try the movement from there.

A bench press is the most popular form of chest press motion. With a bench press, you are positioned flat on your back and just using your chest and arms to press the resistance away from your chest. In a push-up however you are using your core and quads to stabilize your body.

Upper Body
Functional Motions Cont'd

2 CHEST PULL (BACK)

A back pulling motion from the upper body primarily using the back, shoulders, and arms. In this example, we'll be performing a bodyweight pull.

- Start by standing with your feet hip width apart.
- Push your hips and butt backward and let your chest move forward to about a 45 degree angle.
- Extend your arms in front of your chest (downward) to get into the starting position (you would use free weights in your hands when performing this motion in a resistance training workout).
- Bend at the elbows and pull your arms backward until your arms come to a 90 degree angle.

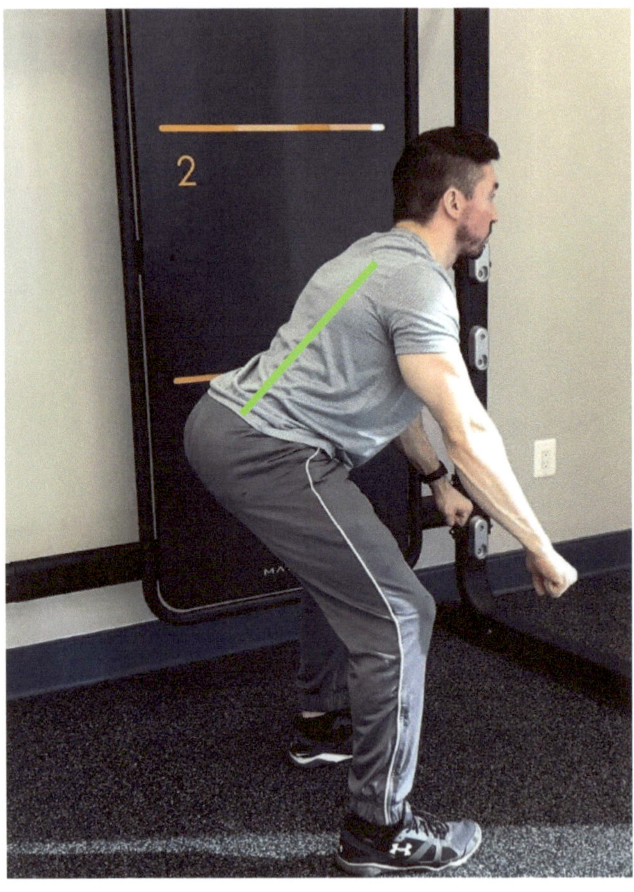
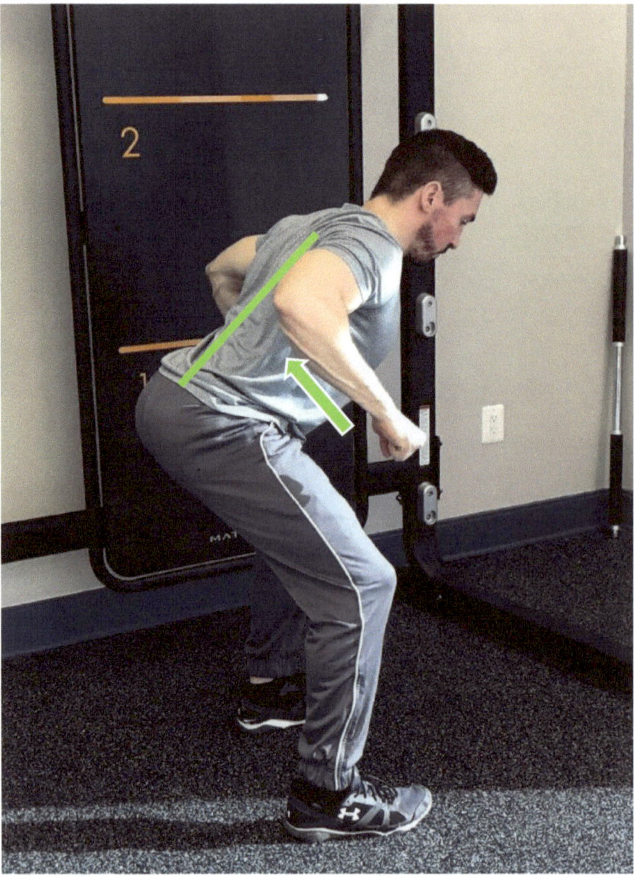

Focus on ensuring your back remains in a straight line (not arched downwards) by keeping your shoulders back and tightening your core through the motion.

Upper Body
Functional Motions Cont'd

3 OVERHEAD PRESS

An upward pressing motion from the upper body primarily using the shoulders, back, and arms. In this example, we'll be performing a bodyweight press.

- Start by standing with your feet about hip width apart.
- Ensure that your back is straight and shoulders are back (good posture).
- Take both hands to shoulder height on either side of your body, bending at the elbows. Your elbows should be directly underneath your hands.
- Press both hands upward and extend your arms into the air.

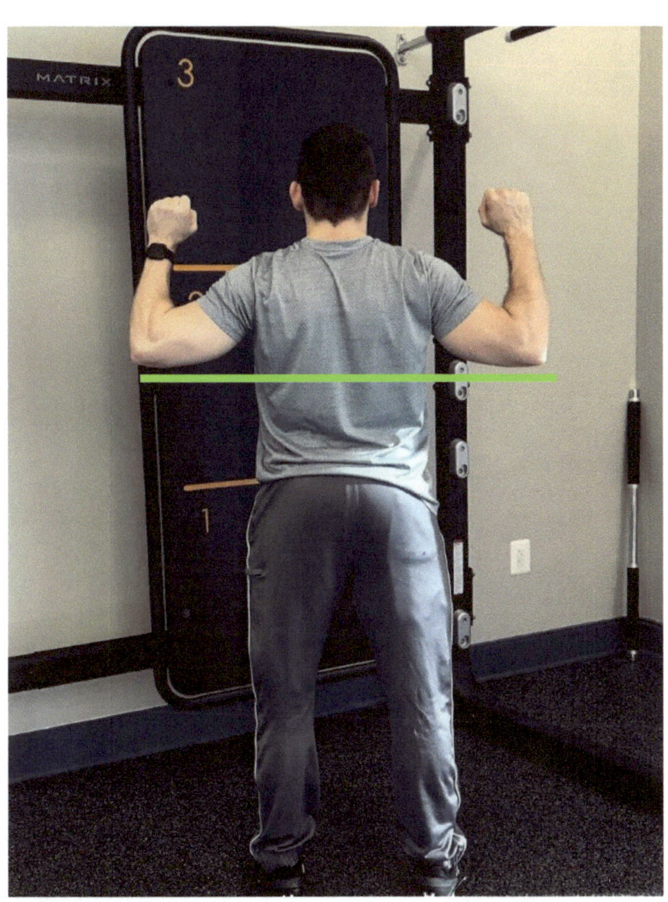
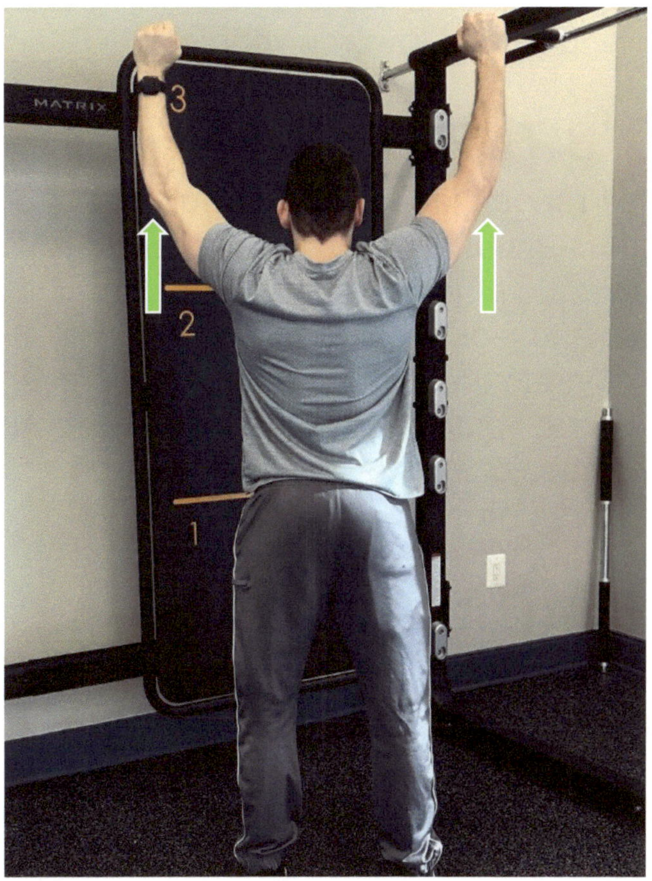

Focus on keeping the arms in a straight line directly above the shoulders. You don't want the arms to go forward or backward when ascending up. During resistance training, you would do this motion with free weights, a barbell, or an assisted machine.

Core / Midsection
Functional Motions

1 CRUNCH

A slight pulling motion for the abdomen. The crunch is isolated to the core.

- Start with your shoulders and back on the ground, with knees bent and feet about hip width apart.
- Take your hands together behind your head (or across your chest).
- Raise your shoulders off of the ground and inward towards your legs.

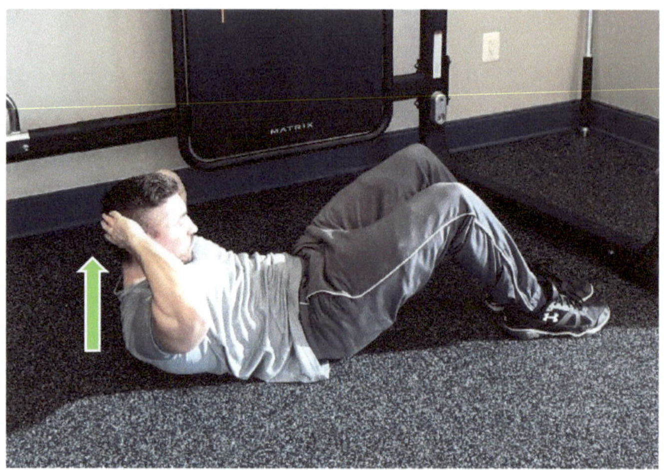

2 SITUP

A full-range motion primarily for the abdomen but also engages other stabilizing muscles in the chest, back, hips, and legs.

- Start in the same position as a crunch.
- Drive your chest upward towards your knees, allowing your full upper body to come off of the ground.

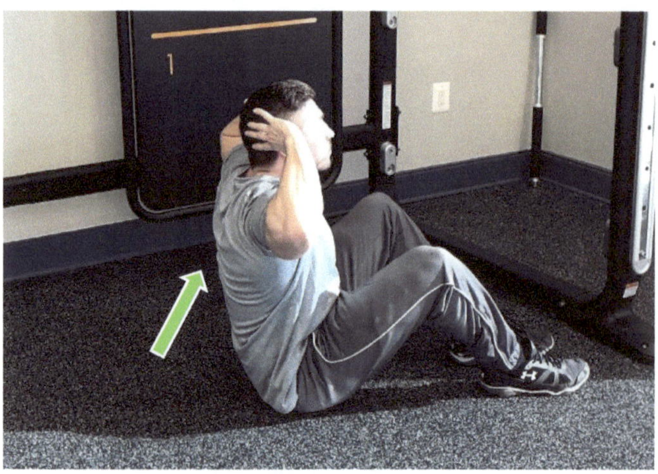

3 SITUP ROTATION

A rotational motion using the torso. A full situp is executed during this motion, in addition to the rotation.

- Start in the same position as a crunch.
- Drive your chest upward towards your knees, but towards the top of the motion, rotate your torso so that the elbow on one side of your body touches the knee on the opposite side of your body.

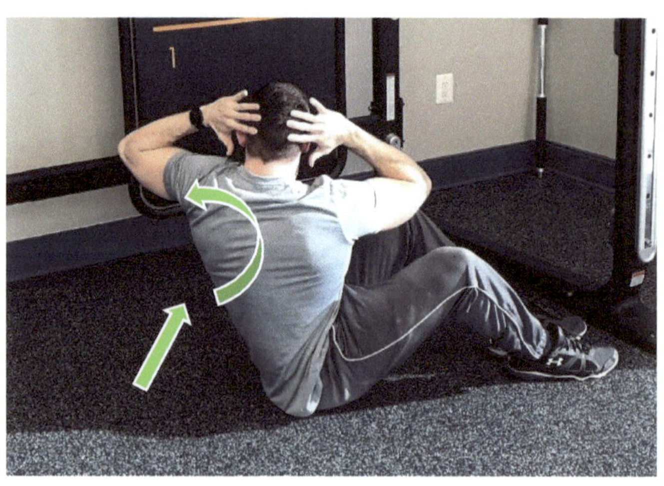

CREATING AND EXECUTING A WORKOUT PLAN

In this section, we'll discuss identifying your current fitness level, setting appropriate goals, tailoring a fitness plan to your individual needs, and executing against that plan.

PHYSICAL ASSESSMENT

Before jumping into exercise, or even starting to set goals, you should first understand your current body composition and fitness level (so you have a baseline):

1. Try out each of the **Primary Functional Movements** (from the previous section) in depth to ensure you have the form nailed down. If any of the movements are difficult to perform, then the form should be worked on before adding any resistance.

2. Take a body composition test – This shouldn't be difficult or expensive. Many nutrition/supplement stores and fitness centers will provide body composition testing for free. We primarily want to identify current bodyfat %:

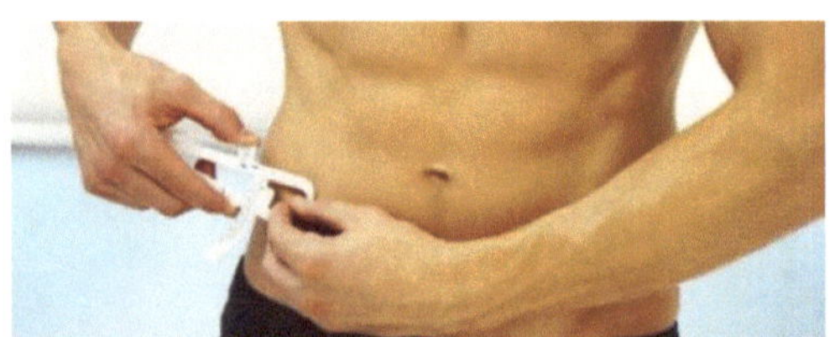

Current Body Composition	
Weight	
Bodyfat %	
Body Type	

Refer to the quick reference guide to see what your bodyfat % means

3. Test yourself on the below exercises:

Running

Time yourself on a 2 mile run and take the average of your mile time (total run time divided by 2).

Great Shape			Good Shape		Average			Out of Shape		Very Out of Shape	
4	5	6	7	8	9	10 mins	11	12	13	14	15

Pushups

Grab a timer and get into position. Here we're going to test how many full-form push-ups you can perform in 60 seconds.

Situps

Similar to the push-up assessment above, let's see how many full-form sit-ups you can perform in 60 seconds.

Use the charts on the next page to see where you stack up on these tests.

PHYSICAL ASSESSMENT

1 Min Pushup Test Ratings

Based on standards published by American College of Sports Medicine (ACSM):

MEN	20-29	30-39	40-49	50-59	60+
Excellent	> 54	> 44	> 39	> 34	> 29
Good	45-54	35-44	30-39	25-34	20-29
Average	35-44	24-34	20-29	15-24	10-19
Poor	20-34	15-24	12-19	8-14	5-9
Very Poor	< 20	< 15	< 12	< 8	< 5

WOMEN	20-29	30-39	40-49	50-59	60+
Excellent	> 48	> 39	> 34	> 29	> 19
Good	34-48	25-39	20-34	15-29	5-19
Average	17-33	12-24	8-19	6-14	3-4
Poor	6-16	4-11	3-7	2-5	1-2
Very Poor	< 6	< 4	< 3	< 2	< 1

Women's standards are based on modified pushups (from knees)

1 Min Situp Test Ratings

Based on standards published by International Fitness Association (IFA):

MEN	20-29	30-39	40-49	50-59	60+
Excellent	>= 47	>= 40	>= 35	>= 30	>= 29
Good	38-46	31-39	25-34	22-29	20-28
Average	34-37	28-30	24-26	19-21	17-19
Below Avg	26-33	21-27	17-23	12-18	10-16
Very Poor	< 26	< 21	< 17	< 12	< 10

WOMEN	20-29	30-39	40-49	50-59	60+
Excellent	>= 37	>= 30	>= 26	>= 21	>= 20
Good	28-36	22-29	18-25	14-20	13-19
Average	25-27	19-21	15-17	11-13	10-12
Below Avg	17-24	12-18	8-14	5-10	4-9
Very Poor	< 17	< 12	< 8	< 5	< 4

GOAL SETTING

Now that you know more about your current body composition and fitness level, you can make smart decisions on your goals.

Setting Your Goals

1. **Start with what you would like to achieve at a high level.**

    Lose weight? Gain muscle mass? Increase endurance? Enhance your balance? Gain energy? Look better naked?

2. **Identify specific, measurable, achievable, realistic goals based on what you want to achieve.**

    If you're goal is to lose weight, you will need to identify your target weight and how long it might take to achieve. A rule of thumb for weight loss is to lose 1-2 lbs per week (as it's more likely to stay off at that rate).

3. **Set a timeline for achieving each individual goal.**

    If you're looking to lose 10 lbs, you could set a target timeline of 5 weeks.

4. **Include milestones (small achievements) along the way**

    Within the example above, you could set milestones for losing 2 lbs each week. These help break up long-term goals into short-term achievements towards the larger goals.

5. **Determine your plan of action for achieving each goal**

    This is the meat of your plan; how you will achieve the outcome. For example, performing moderate cardio 2x per week and resistance training 3x per week.

6. **Identify the best method for tracking your progress.**

    A simple journal (digital or physical) should do the trick.

7. **Make yourself accountable.**

    Tell a friend, coworker or family member about your goals to add a level of accountability, and post the goals somewhere visible to keep them top of mind.

CREATING A WORKOUT PLAN

Developing A Workout Plan

A workout plan should include all of the forms of exercise you plan to complete each week (your weekly regiment), as well as the details of each individual workout. In the beginning of your fitness journey a workout plan should continue for anywhere from 2-12 weeks then change. As you get more experienced, your workout routine may stay relatively consistent for a number of months. The primary indicators of when you should change your workout plan are:

- The workout or exercises within it becomes too easy
- You've hit a plateau and are no longer seeing results

A weekly workout regiment includes:

- Form(s) of exercise you'll perform
- Duration of exercise
- How frequently you'll perform each type of exercise

SAMPLE WEEKLY REGIMENT

- Aerobic: Running
  - 2-3x per week
  - 20-25 minutes

  More cardio than that may reduce muscle mass

- Anaerobic: Resistance Training
  - 3-4x per week
  - 45-60 minutes

  Your body needs lean muscle and movement!

Don't Forget: There is no single workout plan that works for everyone. This will be a trial and error process, but the amount of effort you put in will directly determine your output.

CREATING A WORKOUT PLAN

- Type of exercise(s) to perform
- Duration of exercise
- Level of intensity of the exercise
- If your workout is resistance training based:
    - Which muscle groups are you planning to work (e.g. full body, upper/lower body, or specific individual muscle groups)
    - Which exercises will you perform for those muscle groups
    - What order will you perform the exercises in (biggest motions always come first)
    - What rep and set scheme for each exercise will help you achieve your goal
        - In general, sets of 1-5 reps help with strength/power alone, sets of 6-12 reps help with strength and size, 13+ reps help with muscle definition / body tone.
    - What resistance levels will you use on the exercises
    - What periods of rest will you take during your workout

Workout Focus: Chest Day

Exercise 1: Bench Press (4 Sets)
Set 1 - 10 reps at 50% of max resistance
Set 2 - 10 reps at 60% of max resistance
Set 3 - 8 reps at 65% of max resistance
Set 4 - 6 reps at 70% of max resistance

Exercise 2: Incline Press (3 Sets)
…
Exercise 3: Chest Fly (3 Sets)
…
Exercise 4: Pullover

Make sure overall your workout regiment is comprehensive and well-rounded. You want to develop each side of your body (posterior and anterior equally), and you want to cover aerobic and anaerobic exercise concepts.

EXECUTING A WORKOUT

Before the Workout

Always start with a dynamic warmup, which is active movement (not static stretching). The intention is to get blood flowing to the muscles, open up your joints, and begin to elevate your heart rate.

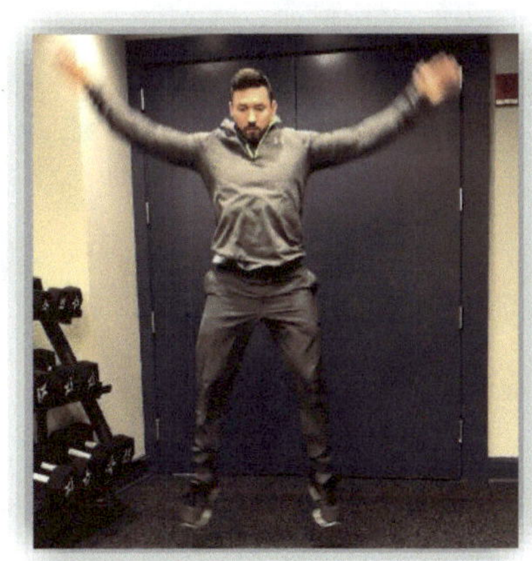

During the Workout

- Start with the largest motions first, the most difficult ones, or the ones that require the most muscle groups (e.g. bench press before bicep curls).

- Perform a warmup of each exercise with bodyweight or light resistance to practice the form before using heavy resistance.

- Breath out through the exercise motion; don't hold your breath.

- Focus (mentally) on the muscles being worked through each motion. A large part of resistance training is the brain telling the right muscles when and how to fire (engage).

- Ensure that each set is challenging to complete. As you get to the last few reps of a set, the motion should be hard to continue. There are several things you can do to increase the challenge level (e.g. increase the resistance, take the motion more slowly to increase the time under tension, increase the intensity of the motion, etc.)

- Don't half-ass any motions. You'll only be cheating yourself.

After the Workout

Rehydrate and replenish your nutrients as soon as possible. Recovery is aided by consumption of nutrients so you'll want to consume nutrients immediately after a workout. Nutrition is a science of its own (which we talk about in our Nutrition Guide), but for starters make sure to get water, electrolytes, and protein immediately after a workout.

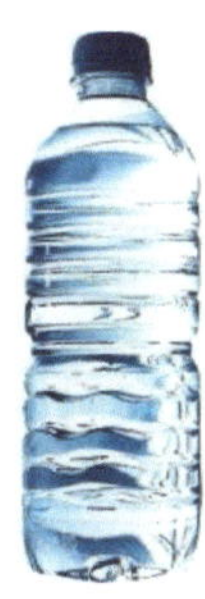

WORKOUTS

You didn't expect me to leave you to create your own workout plans now did you? In this section, I've outlined workout plans for you to get started with.

BACK2BASICS WORKOUT PLANS

In the plans below, I've provided guidance and recommendations for performing each workout plan, however, you should adjust the frequency and duration of the workouts based on your fitness level and goals.

Phase 1: Bodyweight Training and Cardio

In this phase we'll work on functional movements using your bodyweight for resistance. This will start the muscle development process and help perfect form before adding additional resistance.

- **Week 1:** Perform the bodyweight workout 2-3x (spread out across the week) and perform a moderate run 2x (20-30 mins).
- **Week 2:** Perform the bodyweight workout 3-4x (spread out across the week) and perform a moderate run 2x (20-30 mins)

Phase 2: Resistance Training and Cardio

- **Week 3-6+:** Perform the upper body workout 1-2x per week, and the lower body workout 1-2x per week. Ensure that the frequency is equivalent for both muscle groups (i.e. don't perform the upper body workout 2x and the lower body just 1x in a given week). In addition, perform a moderate run 2x per week (20-25 mins).

Example Weekly Plan

Description	Easing Into It	Ready to Work
Monday	Lower Body	Lower Body
Tuesday	Cardio	Upper Body
Wednesday	Rest	Cardio
Thursday	Upper Body	Lower Body
Friday	Cardio	Upper Body
Saturday	Rest	Cardio
Sunday	Rest	Rest

Once you've performed the Phase 2 workout plan for 4+ weeks, you may need to begin adding variety to continue seeing results. You can browse our website for proven workout plans for specific goals.

PHASE 1: BODYWEIGHT

30 Minute Full Body Bodyweight Workout

- Warmup with 20 Jumping Jacks
- Perform each exercise in a circuit below, back to back for the specified number of reps.
- Rest 30-60 seconds before doing the same circuit again for another set / round.
- Perform 3-4 rounds of the same circuit, then head to the next circuit. The finisher round should only be performed once.

Lower Circuit

1 Squat x 15
  Hips back, butt down, drive through heels
2 Forward Lunge x 8 per leg
  Keep shoulders back and chest high
3 Side Lunge x 6 per leg
  Hips back, butt towards heel

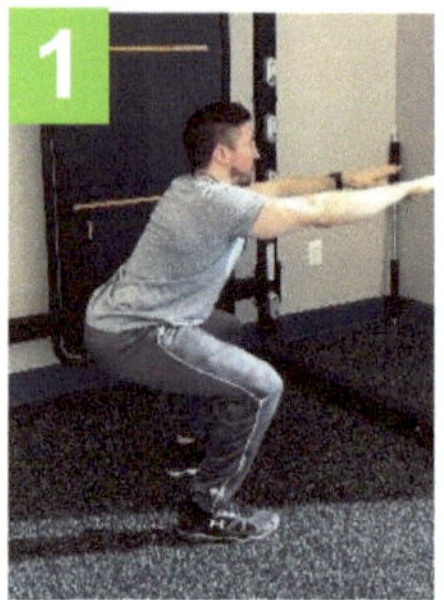 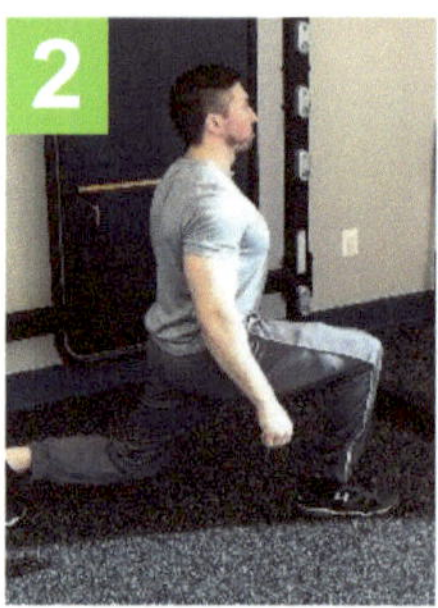 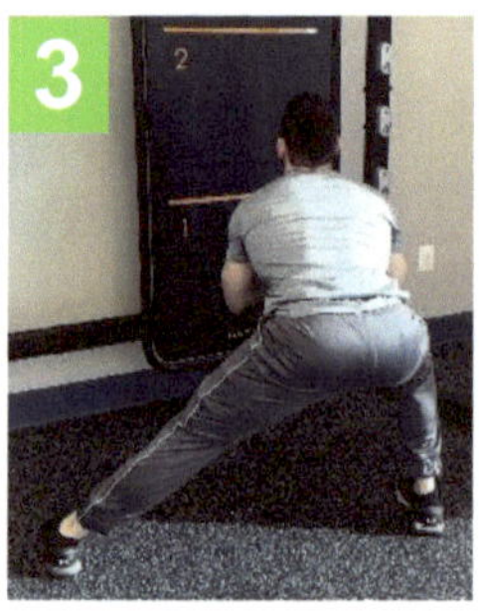

Upper Circuit

1 Pushup x 10
  Try from the knees if needed
2 Plank Rotation x 5 per side
  A wider stance gives more balance
3 Close Grip Pushup x 10
  Hands close together under the chest

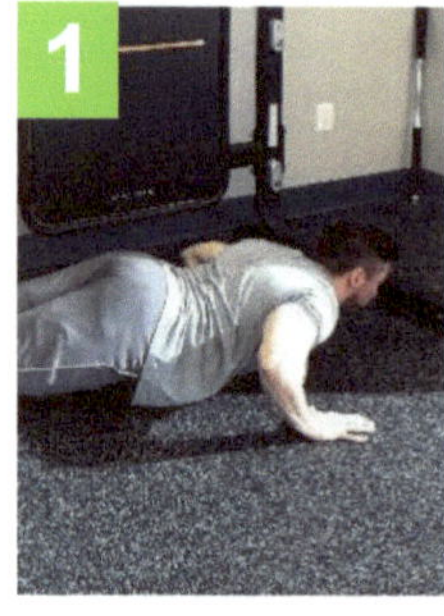 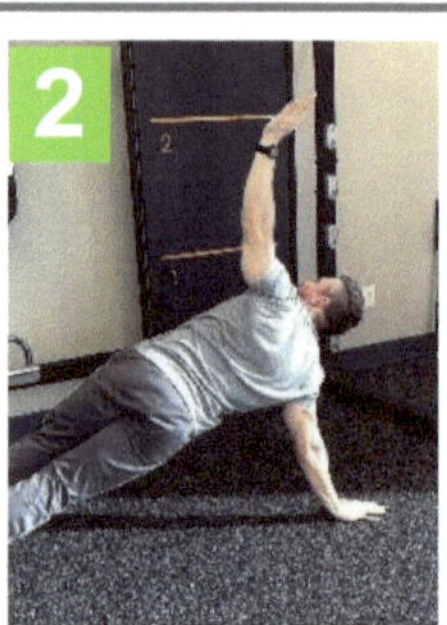 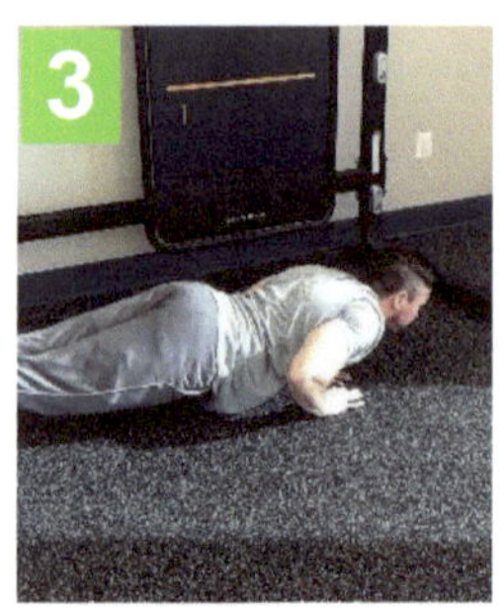

Core Circuit

1 Situp x 10
  Try with hands out front if needed
2 Hip Thrust x 10
  Knees bent, feet flat, drive hips upward
3 Plank Side Tap x 8 per side
  From plank, take one foot to side at a time

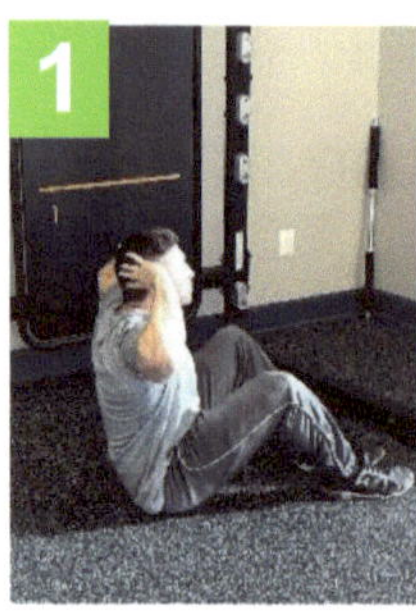 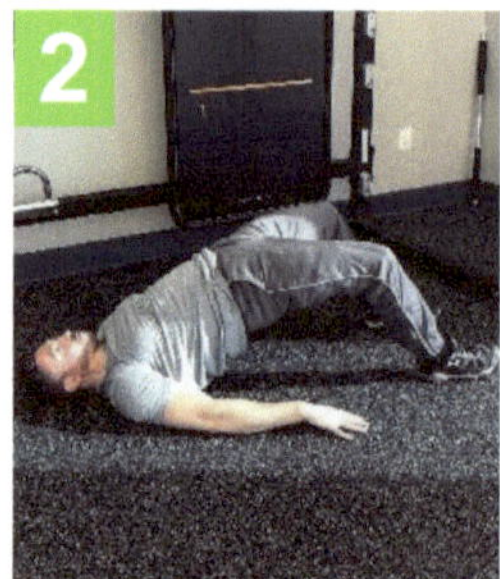 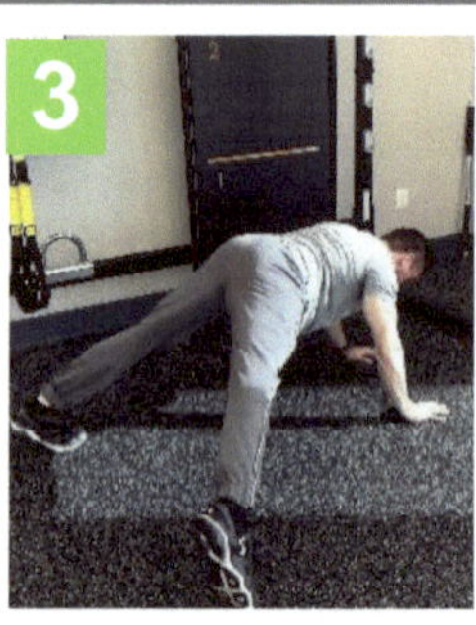

Finishers

1 Squat Jumps x 30 secs
  Squat then jump with power
2 Mountain Climbers x 30 secs
  Bring one knee forward at a time from the high plank (pushup) position

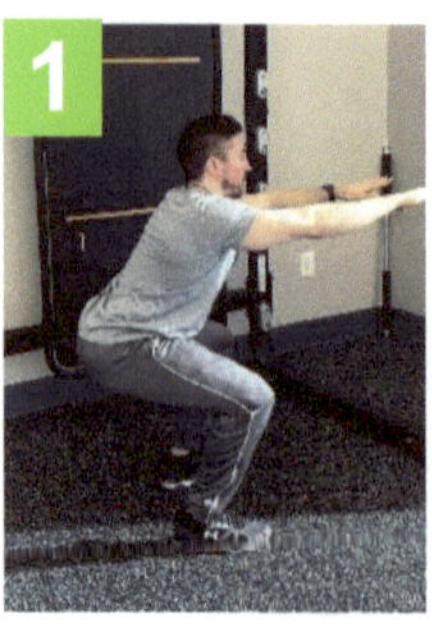 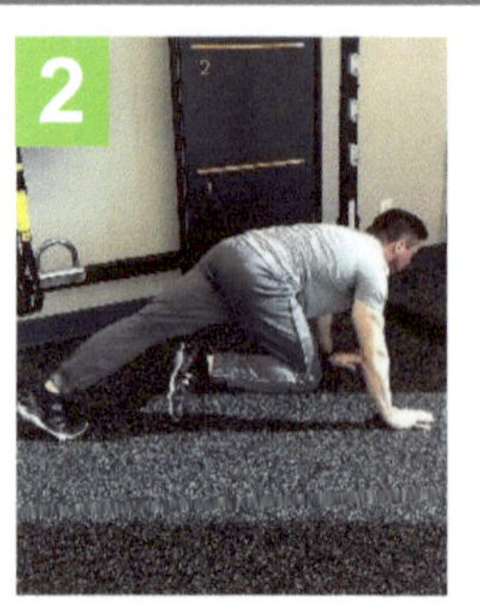

Dynamic Warmup

The following dynamic workout should be performed daily before each resistance training workout.

Windmill x 12

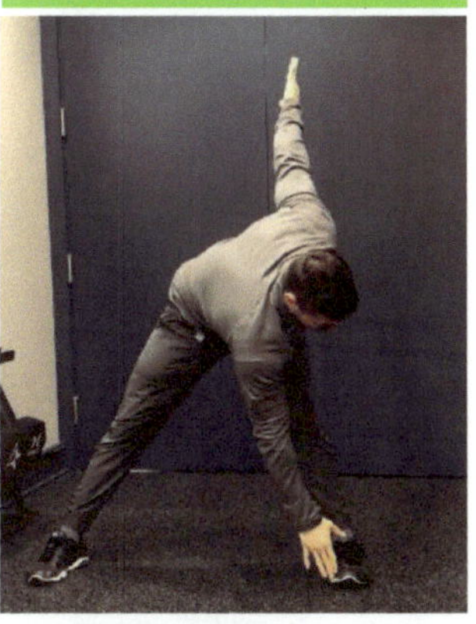

Torso Rotations x 16

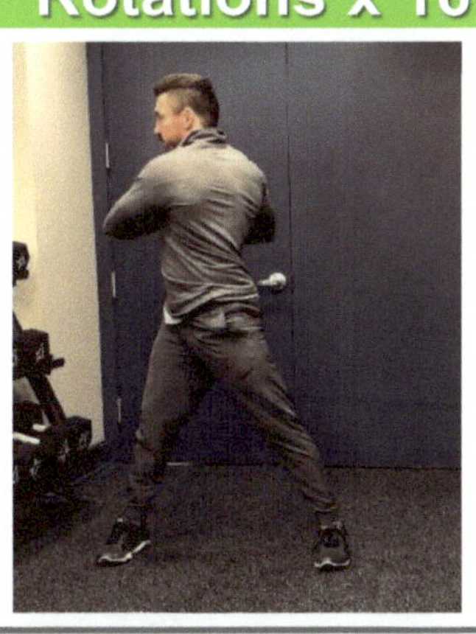

Bodyweight Squats x 10

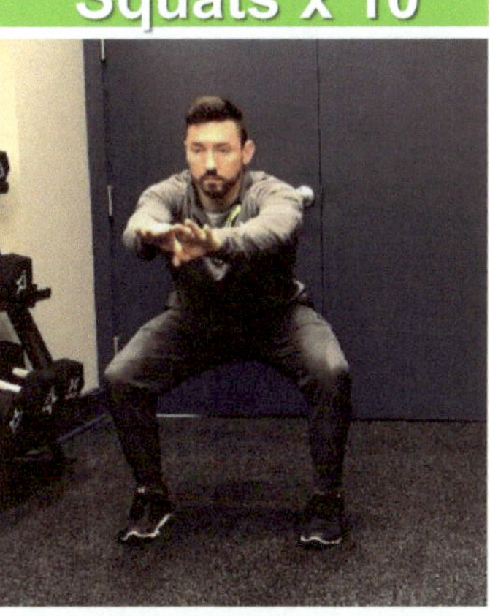

Front Lunges x 5 each

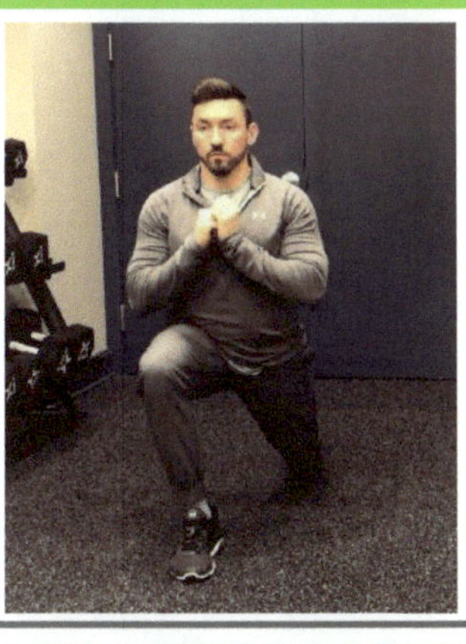

Side Lunges x 5 each

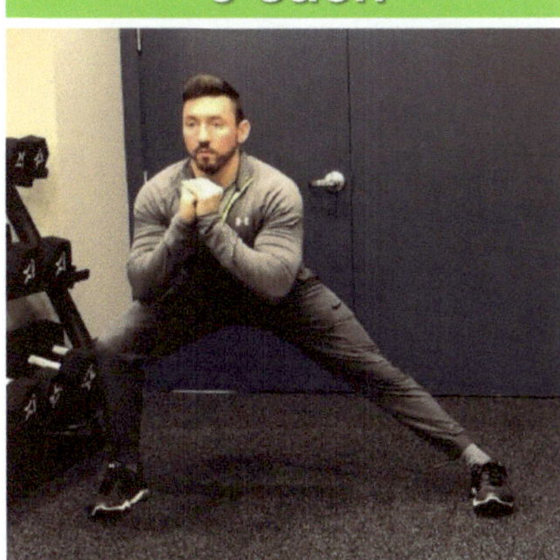

Plank Rotations x 5 each

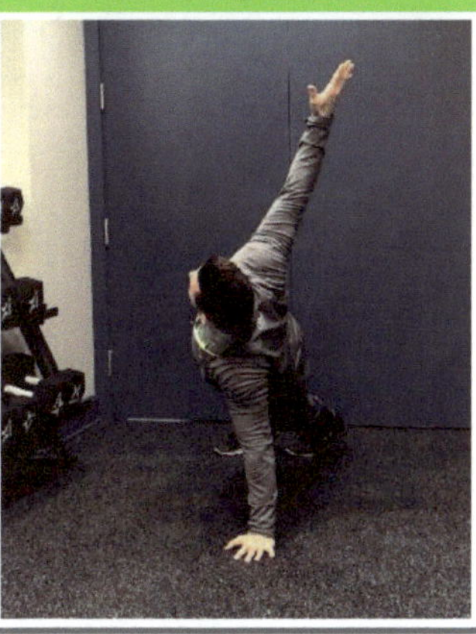

Pushups x 10

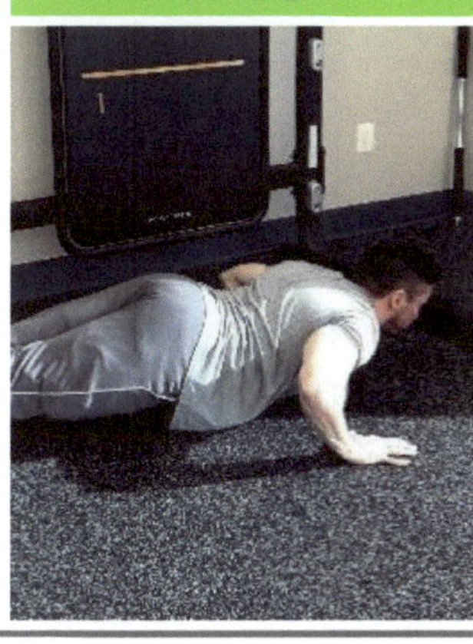

Jumping Jacks x 15

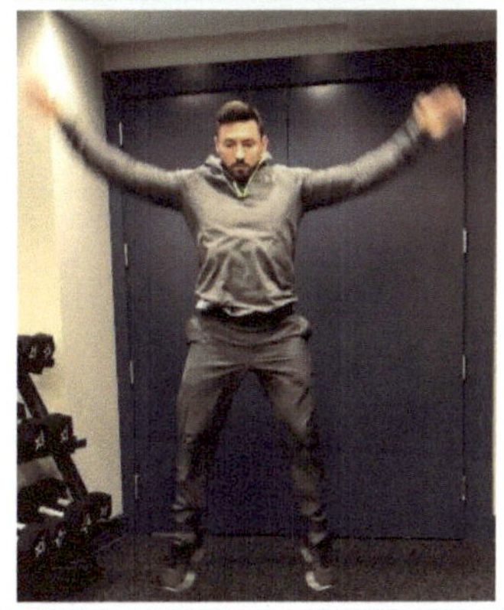

PHASE 2: RESISTANCE

Upper Body Workout

Follow the below exercises in order. Choose a resistance for the first set of each exercise based on what you believe you can complete. Increase the resistance for each set, so that each set is difficult to complete the number of reps. Try to limit your breaks between sets to 60 seconds.

1. Flat Bench Press

- Sets: Warmup x 10, Set 1 x 10, Set 2 x 8, Set 3 x 8, Set 4 x 6
- Dumbbells, Barbell, or Machine Press

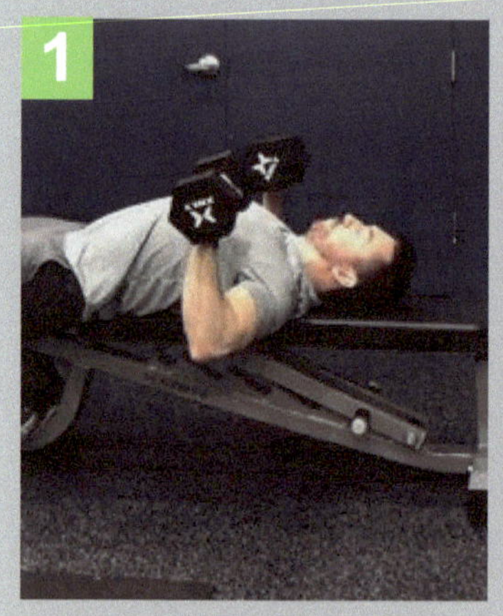
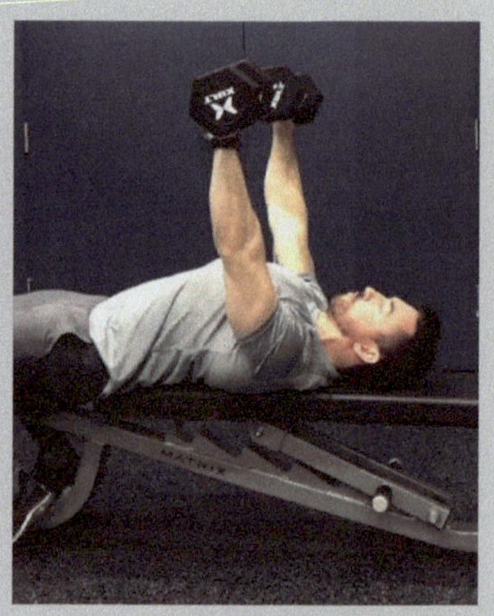

2. Standing Overhead (Shoulder) Press

- Sets: Warmup x 10, Set 1 x 10, Set 2 x 8, Set 3 x 8, Set 4 x 6
- Dumbbells, Barbell, or Machine Press

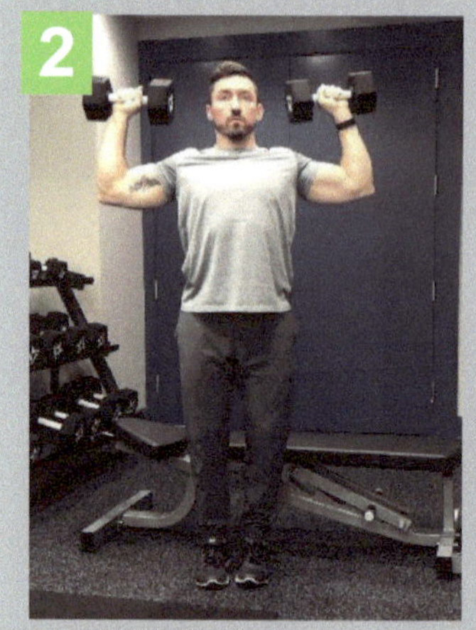
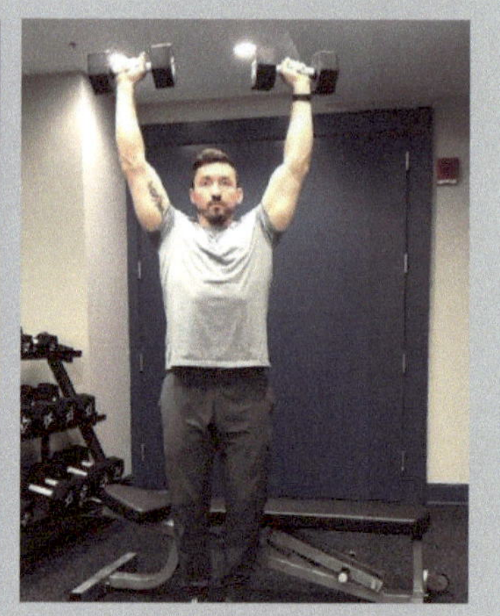

3. Lat Pull Down (or Pullups)

- Sets: Set 1 x 12, Set 2 x 10, Set 3 x 10, Set 4 x 8
- Lat Pull Down Machine or Pullup Bar

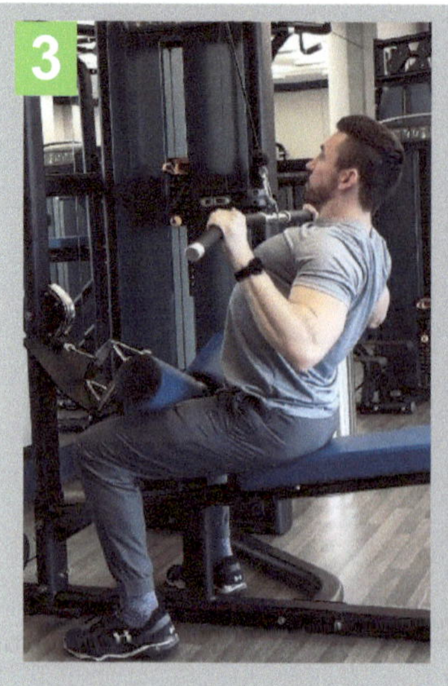
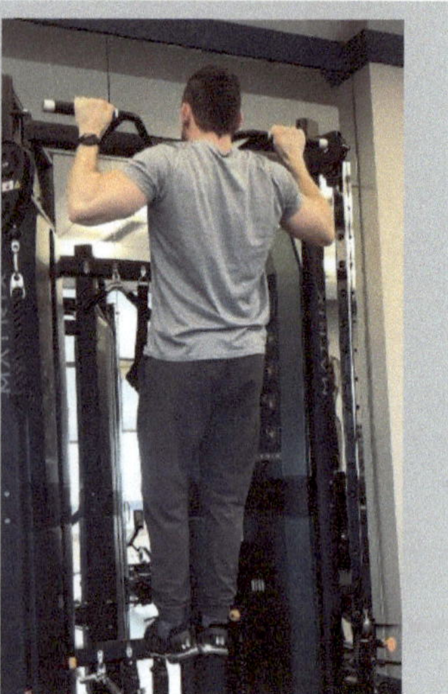

PHASE 2: RESISTANCE

Upper Body Workout Con'td

4. Single Arm Row

- Sets: Set 1 x 10 each, Set 2 x 8 each, Set 3 x 6 each
- Dumbbells or Barbell

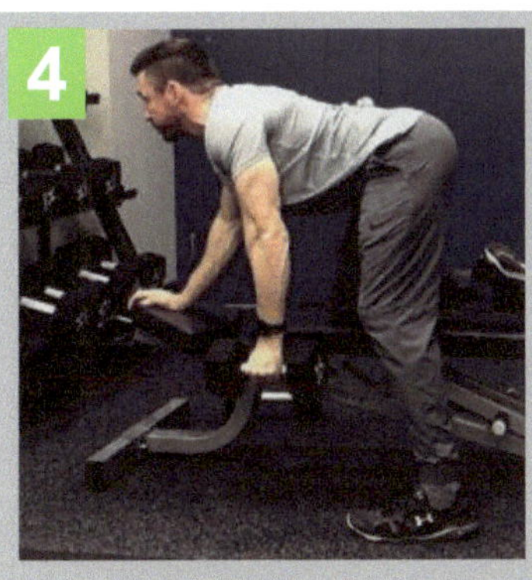
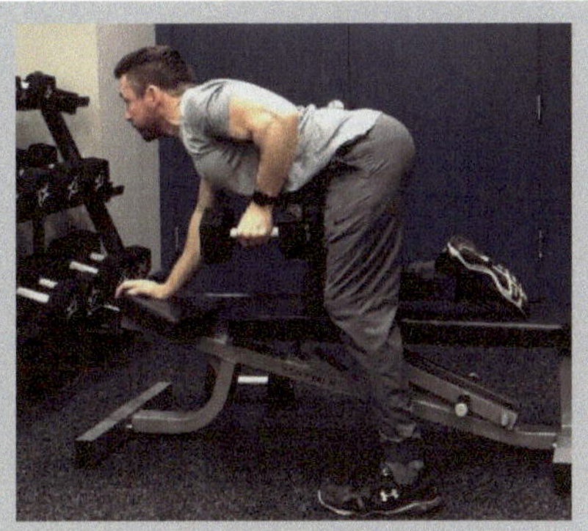

5. Superset: Side Raise and Chest Fly

- Perform 1 set of Side Raises followed by 1 set of Chest Flys, break then perform the 2nd set.
- Sets: Set 1 x 10, Set 2 x 10, Set 3 x 8
- Dumbbells

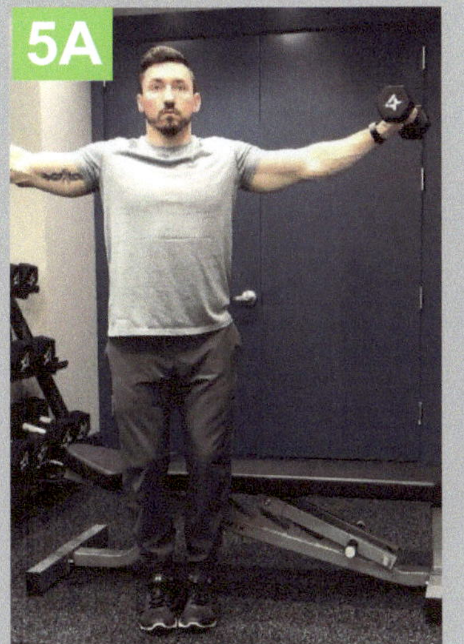
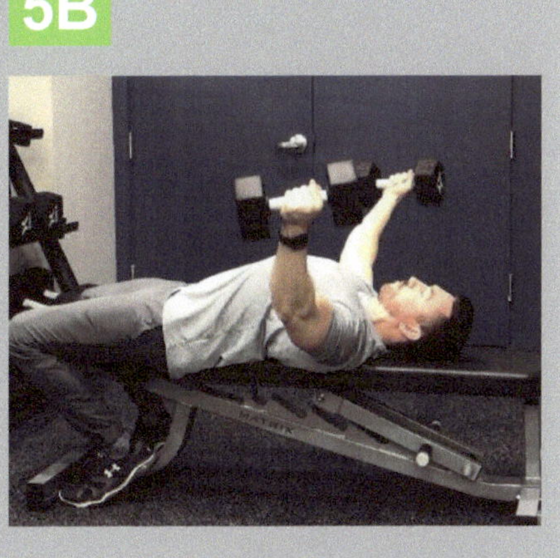

6. Superset: Bicep Curl and Tricep Extension

- Perform 1 set of Bicep Curls followed by 1 set of Tricep Extension, break then perform the 2nd set.
- Sets: Set 1 x 15, Set 2 x 12, Set 3 x 10
- Dumbells

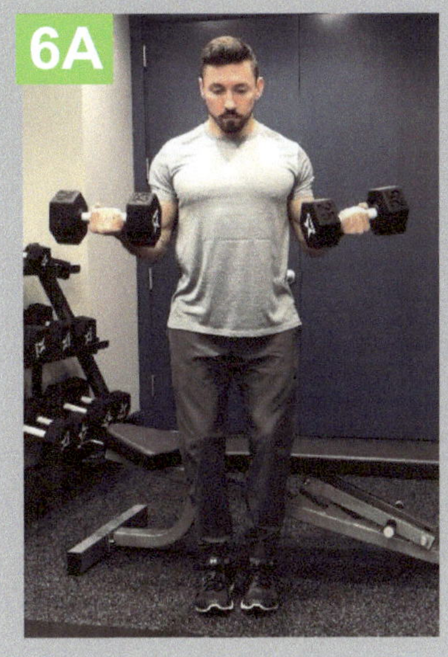
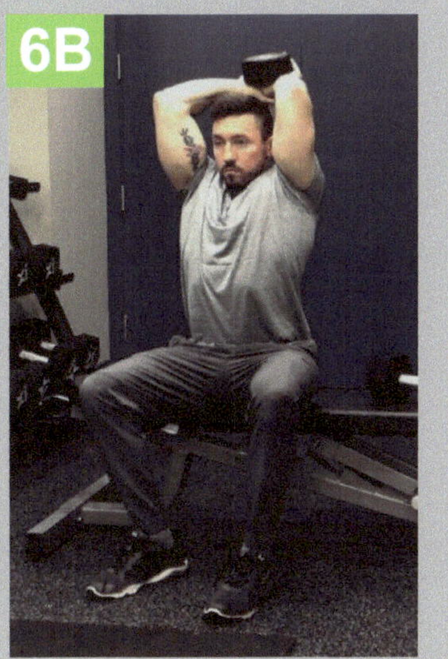

Lower Body Workout

Follow the below exercises in order. Choose a resistance for the first set of each exercise based on what you believe you can complete. Increase the resistance for each set, so that each set is difficult to complete the number of reps. Try to limit your breaks between sets to 60 seconds.

1. Squat

- Sets: Warmup x 10, Set 1 x 10, Set 2 x 8, Set 3 x 8, Set 4 x 6
- Dumbbells, Barbell, or Smith Machine

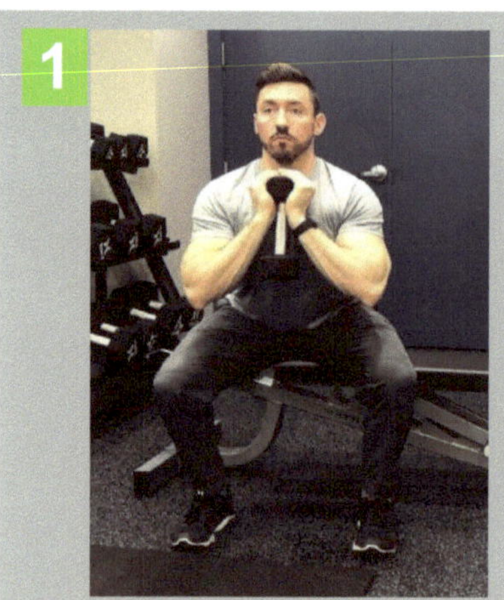
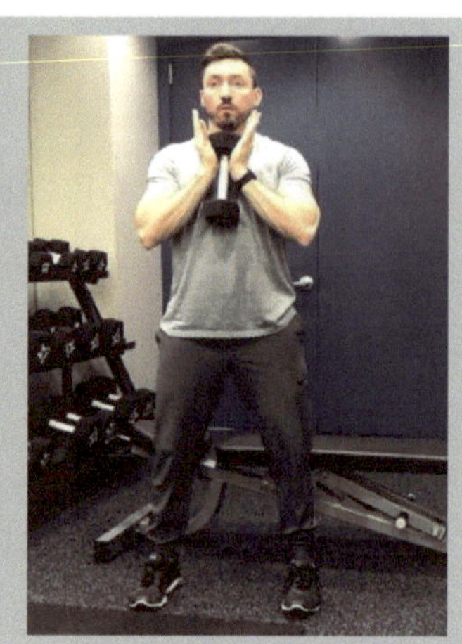

2. Forward Lunge

- Sets: Set 1 x 8 each, Set 2 x 8 each, Set 3 x 6 each
- Dumbbells or Barbell

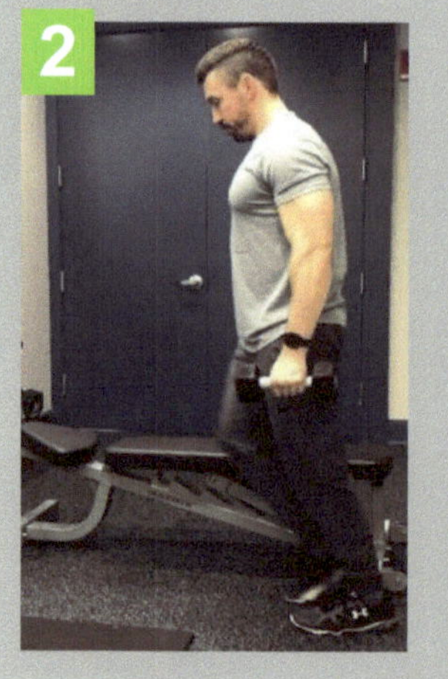
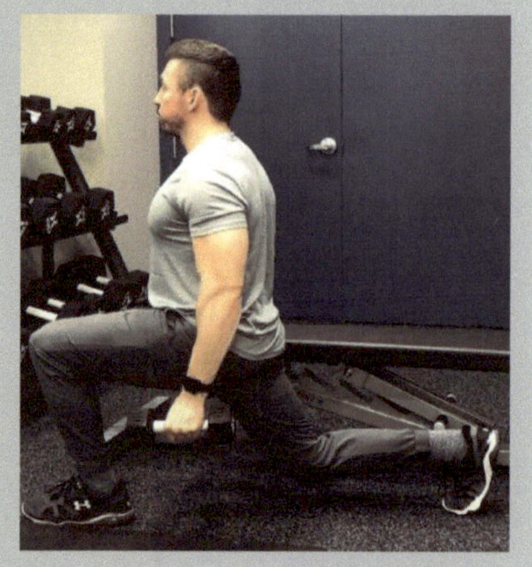

3. Bench Step Up

- Sets: Set 1 x 8 each, Set 2 x 8 each, Set 3 x 6 each
- Dumbbells

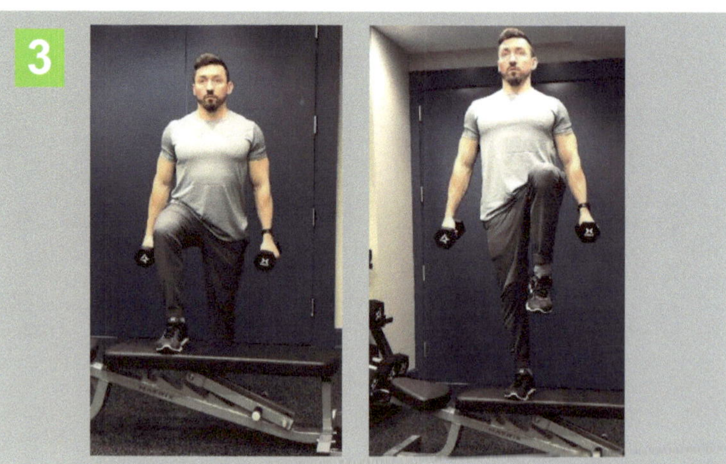

Lower Body Workout Cont'd

4. Hamstring Curl

- Sets: Set 1 x 12, Set 2 x 10, Set 3 x 8, Set 4 x 8
- Hamstring Curl Machine or Resistance Band

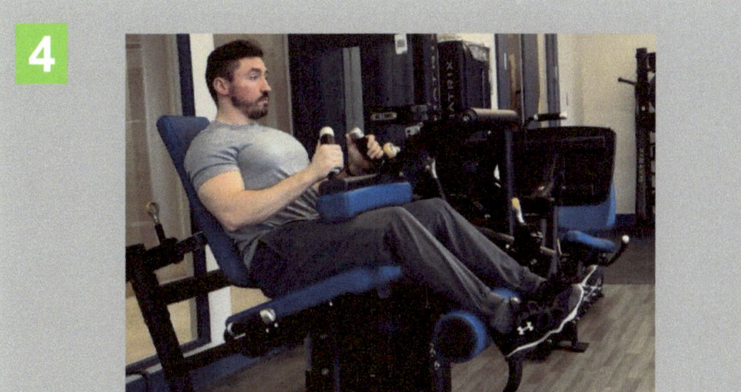

5. Leg Extension

- Set 1 x 12, Set 2 x 10, Set 3 x 8, Set 4 x 8
- Leg Extension Machine or Resistance Band

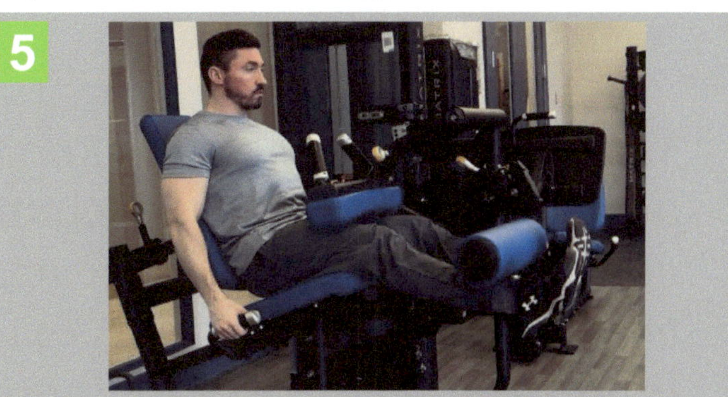

6. Calf Raise

- Set 1 x 20, Set 2 x 16, Set 3 x 12
- Dumbbells or Calf Raise Machine

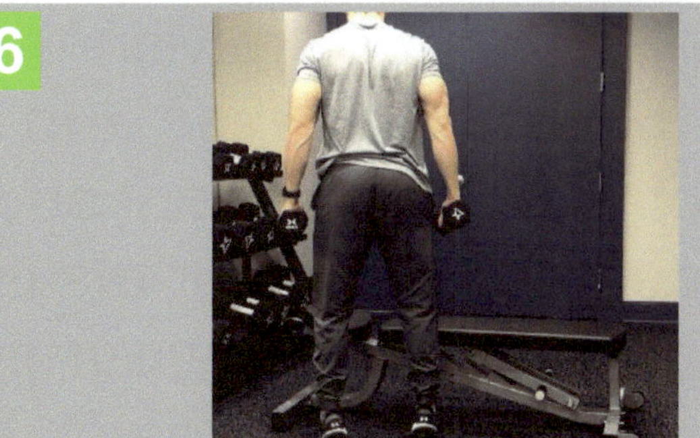

7. Squat Jumps

- Set 1 x 30 secs, Set 2 x 20 secs, Set 3 x 15 secs
- Bodyweight

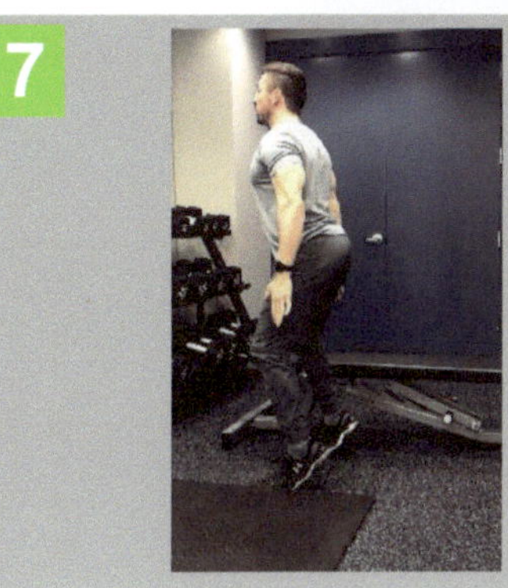
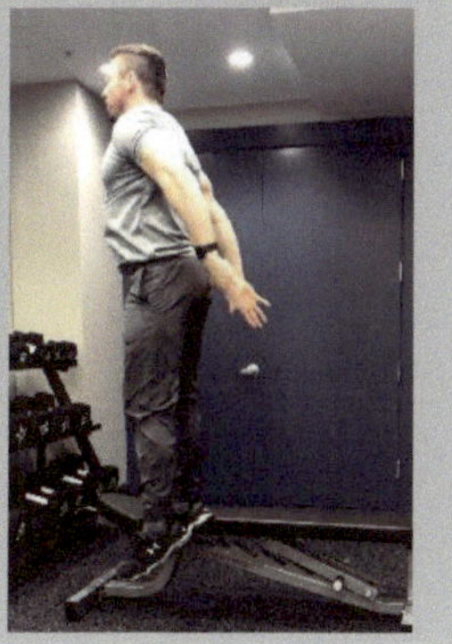

YOU CAN DO THIS!

Everyone has to start somewhere, and by readying this guide you're already ahead of the game. Just taking the step to get active is an achievement, but don't forget that the effort you put in will directly correlate to the benefits you get out of exercise.

Exercise doesn't have to be hard and it certainly doesn't have to be daunting. Go into an exercise plan with a positive mindset, focus on what you want to achieve, and have some fun with it. You'll never regret investing in your health!

Quick Tips For A Successful Health Journey:

- **Take baby steps**. Don't jump right in to the most challenging actions possible. Your much more likely to succeed and keep consistent healthy habits if you incorporate small changes at a time until they become a habit.
- **Incorporate accountability to stick to your plan** (e.g. put your plan somewhere visible, invite a friend in on the fun)
- **Monitor your progress and track your success**. If you take note of your starting point and your milestones, you'll be able to better recognize your results.
- **Compare yourself to your previous self, not to others.** Everyone's body is different. Work on making a better you; a you that is better than you were the previous day.

Now, let's get to work!

THE END

Thank you for reading!
Don't forget to stop by our website to browse additional guides, workout plans, and more to keep your body in tip-top shape!

www.ingramcontent.com/pod-product-compliance
Lightning Source LLC
Chambersburg PA
CBHW040148240726
48664CB00002B/636